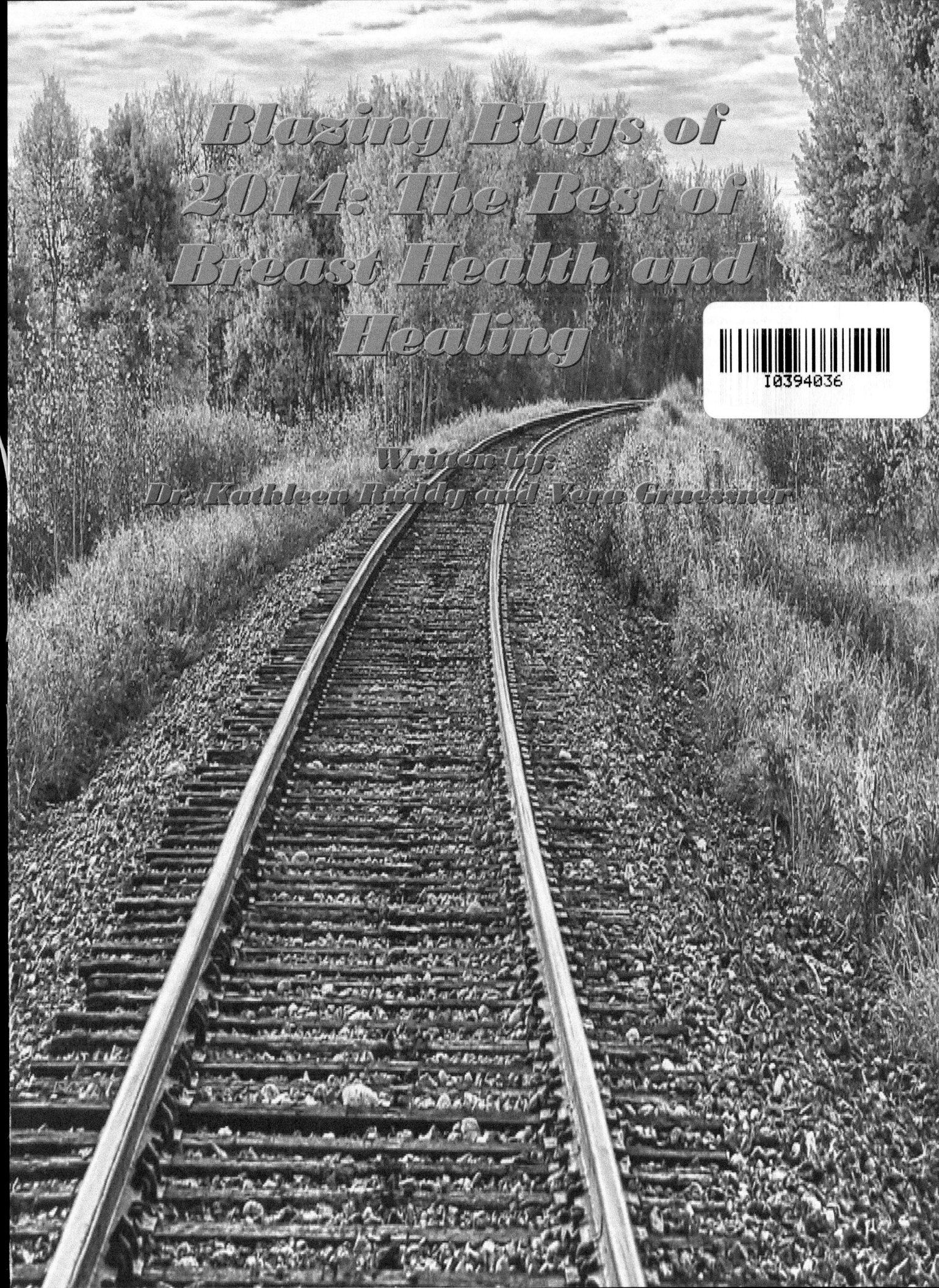

Introduction

This anthology of blogs from the Breast Health and Healing Foundation will help you in a variety of ways. Whether you are a breast cancer patient, a caregiver, a cancer survivor, at high risk of the disease, or solely a woman, this book will provide a wide variety of information that will help you learn more about breast cancer and ways to prevent it.

The anthology goes over the symptoms of breast cancer, diagnostics, treatments and medications, important cancer research projects, and vital prevention tactics such as favorable nutrition and fitness.

By learning key details in the fight against breast cancer, you will gain the ability to reduce your risk of this disease. Be sure to let friends and family know about the research on the breast cancer virus and the multitude of prevention techniques provided in this book. The breast cancer virus and preventive vaccine are vital areas of science research that may bring a "pure cure" to this disease once and for all.

This book was put together to offer our regular blog readers and women around the country a superb collection of some of the best articles we've created over the last year. It was formed to help women prevent this disease and/or find the best treatments in order to survive cancer. Essentially, this book was created to save lives!

Our anthology is full of tips and facts that will help you learn about the diagnostics, treatments, and prevention of breast cancer. We invite you to read the best blogs we've written over the last year. And don't forget to share this book with your loved ones!

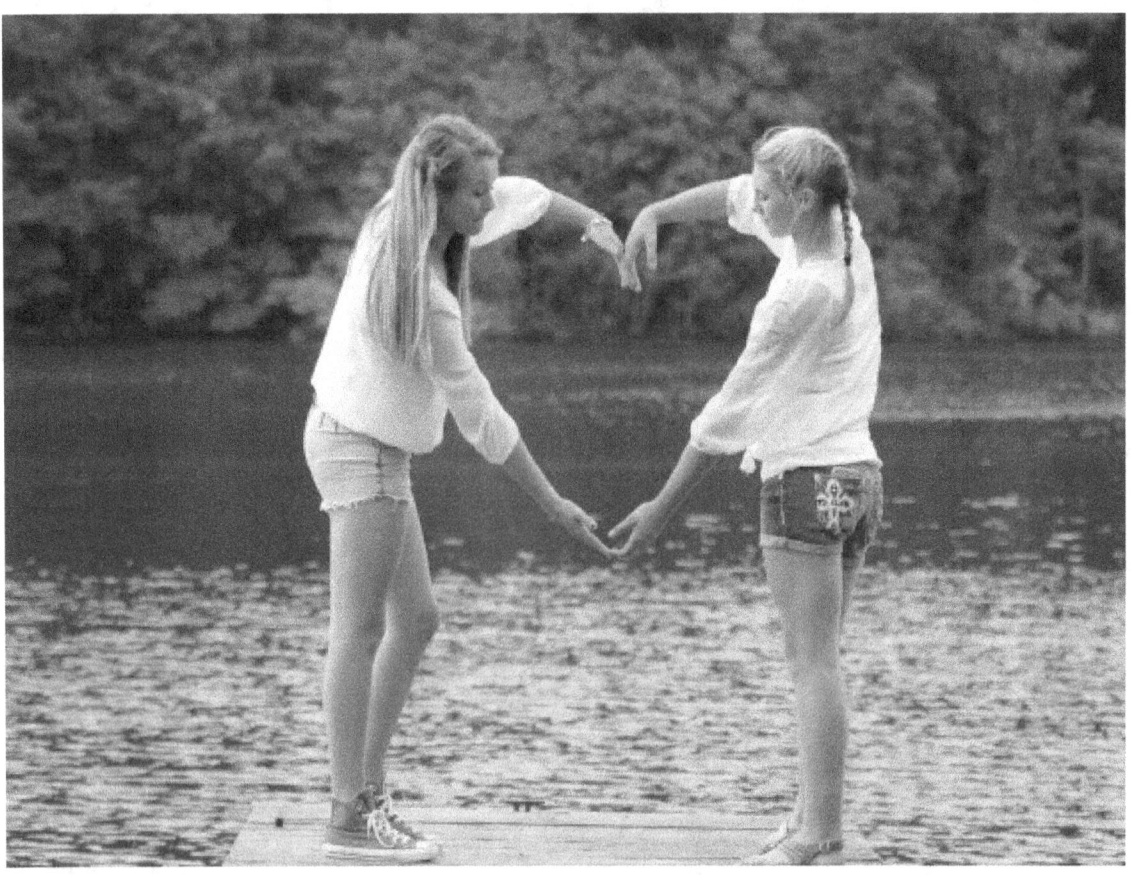

5. Manage your worst symptoms with your doctor - you don't have to suffer!

6. Talk to other cancer survivors to gather more support and advice.

Common Causes of Burning in the Breast

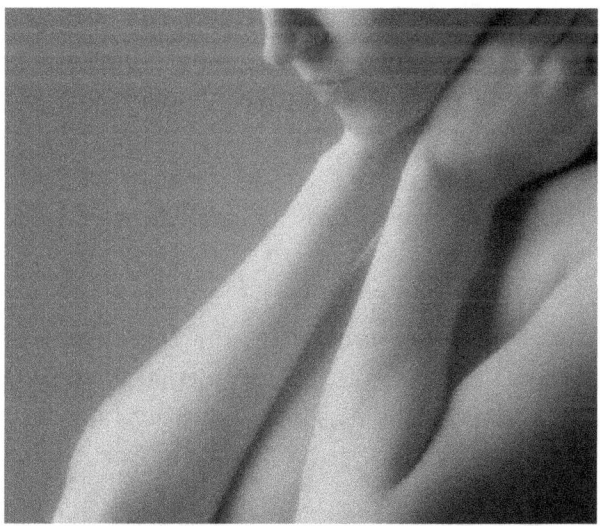

Burning breast pain can be felt in one or both breasts. The breast includes complex system of glandular tissues, blood vessels, lymph nodes as well as connective nerves and tissues. Some of the primary causes of burning breast pains are damaged breast tissue and pinched or irritated nerves. While 90 percent of breast pain is not associated with cancer, it is recommended to consult the case to a physician to erase any suspicion and to have a thorough evaluation.

Fatty Acid

What we eat affects not only our stomach but the whole body as well. Burning sensation can be well attributed to dairy products. It may be due to how the body breaks down the fats or the animal's hormone. Due to these reasons, fatty acid imbalance influences the sensitivity of breast tissues.

Stress

Stress, in any form, does not have good effect on the body. Emotions, immune system, and hormone directly affect each other. Because everyone has a different level of stress tolerance and stressors, the burning sensation will also vary in its manifestation.

EDITOR'S TIP:

Life after Breast Cancer: The Next Steps Post Recovery

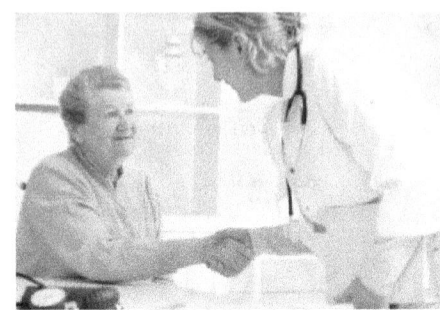

Eight months ago, you felt a lump during your monthly self-exam. You went to see your doctor who scheduled you for a biopsy. After several tests, your physician told you that your left breast had a malignant tumor. You underwent all of the chemotherapy, surgery, and other assigned procedures to fight your cancer and come out on the other side.

Yesterday, the oncologist said that you are now cancer-free. Tears of joy filled your eyes. You couldn't be happier. You're a survivor! Now what?

Even if you overcame this disease, life will not be the same. It never is. Instead of returning to your life as it once was, you will have to get used to a "new normal." WebMD explains that some of the biggest issues you will have to tackle as a breast cancer survivor is the side effects of treatment. You will need to take time to recover from the battle your body has just been through.

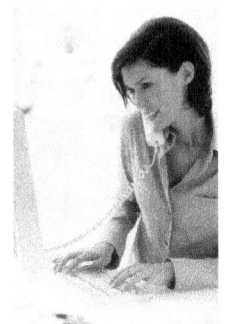

You're likely to still feel significantly tired and experience "chemobrain," which may include the inability to focus and some memory lapses. It may take the same amount of time as treatment itself did before you begin feeling closer to your old self.

You must understand that even though treatment is over, you will not be able to jump right back into your old lifestyle. Your boss and co-workers need to know that you won't be able to sit in on all of the same conferences and meet the strictest deadlines because of your ongoing fatigue. Your children's schools need to know you won't be able to participate in the same car pools and bake sales as usual. The Fred Hutchinson Cancer Research Center provides ten tips for breast cancer survivors to follow after treatment. Below is an outline of some of these recommendations.

1. Have a brief overview of your breast cancer treatments.

2. Talk to your doctor about monitoring your long-term side effects of treatment.

3. Keep exercising and moving to lower your risk of cancer recurrence.

4. Eat a diet of whole grains, vegetables, and fruits.

Breast pain disappears after several weeks or month, but if you cannot tolerate the pain anymore, pain relievers are available over the counter to deal with the pain. Sometimes, a simple brassiere can be the culprit. Using an appropriately sized bra will help support the breast, because there are days when it is sensitive. Excessive fat consumption, salty foods, caffeine and alcohol intake can also lead to this condition. Do various relaxation treatments to control the nervousness of being in breast pain. If the burning persists, consulting a physician will help alleviate the problem and trace down its cause.

Nerve Pressure

This non-cyclic pain is due to a pinched nerve from the cervical or back area. Muscoskelatal history like arthritis, back injury, or osteoporosis is linked to breast pain.

Medication Used

Hormone replacement therapy and birth control pills also causes breast pain due to the hormones included in them. The pills' hormones can contribute to the body's own hormone production, which can cause an imbalance.

Reproductive Hormones

Breast pain for women is largely related to monthly menstrual cycle. Some women produce little or too much estrogen while others have low progesterone level. This hormonal flux causes throbbing pains, which is termed as cyclical breast pain. This is not related to breast cancer and frequently diminishes on menopausal period. To ease the pain, sufferers can purchase over the counter medicines like ibuprofen, gel pain relievers, or paracetamol.

Burning breast pains that causes momentary twinge should not be ignored. The throbbing ache might be a symptom of a serious illness. It is best to consult a doctor to know the underlying condition and to seek proper prevention steps. Aside from physical examination, patients can also undergo a series of tests to ensure that the burning sensation is not associated with any form of serious cases or sickness. Remember that disregarding it can lead to serious complications and higher health risks.

Huge News: The Affordable Care Act Dictates Insurance Cover Breast Cancer Prevention Drugs

The Obama administration's Patient Protection and Affordable Care Act has brought significant changes to the healthcare system in this country. Young adults, for instance, are now allowed to stay on their parents' health insurance plans until they reach 26 years of age. Insurance

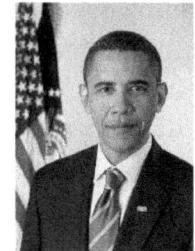

companies can no longer claim proper health insurance from people with pre-existing conditions. Preventive services have also gained ground.

A new service that the Obama administration has issued is requiring insurance companies to cover the costs of the breast cancer drugs tamoxifen and raloxifene, according to Time Magazine. The U.S. Preventive Services Task Force uncovered recently that these drugs are able to prevent breast cancer in women who are at high-risk.

Because the Affordable Care Act includes clauses that require insurance to cover preventive care, these drugs will be covered by health insurance companies without putting any other costs onto female patients.

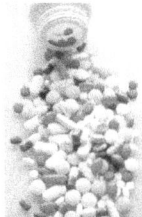
"We've known that we can reduce the risk of breast cancer for women at high risk. But despite the knowledge and availability there is little traction in the clinical and patient community," Dr. Len Lichtenfeld, the deputy chief medical officer of the American Cancer Society, told the source. ""For some women, the question may have been cost and affordability. For that segment of the population, this might make a difference."

This new approach to breast cancer prevention for high-risk women will be taken care of by the insurance companies along with preventive screening methods. High-risk women are also covered for breast cancer genetic testing and the doctor consultation of the results.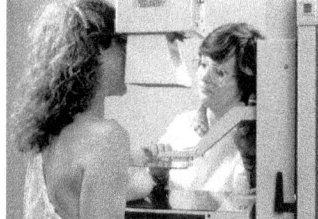

This is truly wonderful news for those who've seen close family members battle the disease. If you've seen your mother or grandmother struggle with breast cancer, you should know that your daughters and nieces will have a higher chance of preventing this disease due to the Affordable Care Act.

Along with taking the appropriate medication, women at high-risk of breast cancer should also exercise regularly, eat a plant-based diet, abstain from smoking and excessive alcohol, and evade hormone replacement therapy (HRT).

Yoga & Its Benefits: It May Reduce Inflammation & Fatigue in Breast Cancer Survivors

Breast cancer survivors are often stuck overcoming a multitude of side effects of treatment for months or years after their medical care ends. One major problem is fatigue. Women are often left feeling exhausted, which is troublesome when work deadlines are looming, children need attention, or family obligations are impending.

Luckily, a new study stemming from Ohio State University shows that yoga may help reduce the fatigue and sleeping troubles of breast cancer survivors after they have undergone treatments like chemotherapy or radiation, according to Health Day News. The study was published in the January edition of *"The Journal of Clinical Oncology."* As many as 60 percent of breast cancer survivors also claim to have trouble sleeping, which may be adding to the fatigue they feel.

"Even some years out from breast cancer treatment, anywhere from 30 to 40 percent of women report substantial levels of fatigue," study author Janice Kiecolt-Glaser, a professor of psychology and psychiatry at Ohio State University, told the source.

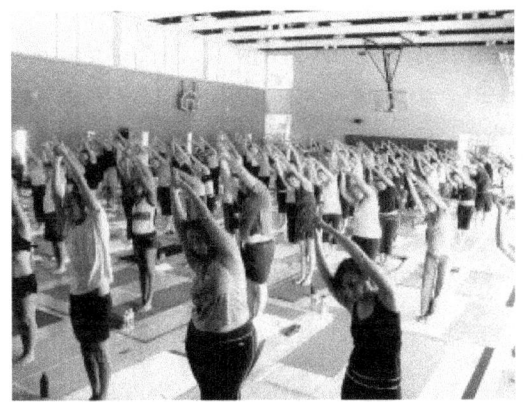

Kiecolt-Glaser and her colleagues gathered 200 women between age 27 to 76 as subjects for their study on whether yoga can alleviate fatigue. All of these women had been survivors for three years or less. Half of the women were recruited to participate in Hatha yoga for two 90-minute sessions every week. The rest were left as a control group.

After three months, the women taking yoga reported they were feeling more alive and were sleeping better. After six months, they were feeling 60 percent less fatigue than the women in the control group. Additionally, the measurements of their inflammation were 13 to 20 percent lower than those not practicing yoga. The Boston Globe reported that these women had 20 percent lower levels of proteins that are markers for inflammation circulating the cardiovascular system. Excess inflammation has been linked with breast cancer recurrence, heart disease, osteoporosis, and diabetes. Clearly, anything that lowers inflammation should be incorporated into your weekly routine!

"It's pretty consistent now across a number of different studies that yoga can be useful for improving symptoms like fatigue and sleep disturbances, which are extremely prevalent in breast cancer survivors and cancer survivors, in general," Lorenzo Cohen, director of the integrative medicine program at M.D. Anderson Cancer Center in Houston, told Health Day News.

Whether you are a breast cancer survivor or just looking to stay healthy, you may want to consider incorporating yoga into your life. It could prevent health issues and keep you more vibrant!

What is the TNM Breast Cancer Staging System?

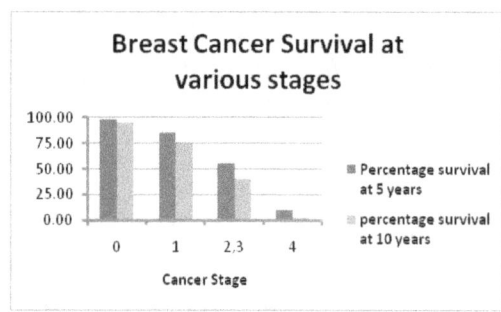

The word stage usually refers to what extent something has progressed. Breast cancer progresses in stages. Each stage describes what is happening to the body, and to what level the cancer has spread. During treatment of breast cancer, the stage of the cancer is one of the determining factors. The Tumor Node Metastasis (TNM) staging system is the standard used to measure breast cancer malignancy that has been in use for treatment of breast cancer.

How is Breast Cancer Staging Done?

The staging of breast cancer is performed by the use of imaging tests such as mammograms, computed tomography (CT) scans, chest x-rays, and magnetic resonance imaging (MRI). In addition to these, physical exams and biopsies also help doctors evaluate breast cancer stages. Lastly, blood tests are sometimes performed to indicate general health of the patient, as well as show if the cancer has spread to other parts of the body.

Who Came up With the TNM System?

The TNM staging system was developed more than 60 years ago by Pierre Denoix of France, but wasn't applied to breast cancer until the late 1960s. After its introduction, the American Joint Committee on Cancer (AJCC) improved upon the first model and made it a standardized way for cancer doctors to evaluate the extent of the disease in patients.

A BRIEF HISTORY

The TNM system was developed between 1943 and 1952 by Pierre Denoix as a classification system for malignant tumors. In 1953, a World Health Organization Sub-Committee on Cancer Registration and Presentation agreed on the staging system, and since then has been adopted worldwide as the standard for describing and classifying cancer progression stages.

How is Breast Cancer Malignancy Classified?

By using the TNM staging system, breast cancer malignancy is classified according to the T, N, and M stages. The letter T takes into account the size of the cancerous tumor, N determines whether the cancer has affected the lymph nodes, and M indicates if the cancer has spread to other body organs. The letter T usually has a number in the 0-4 range that indicates the size of the tumor and how far it is under the breast. The letter N has a number in the 0-1 range that shows the number of lymph nodes affected, and M has 0 or 1 to show if body organs are affected.

How do They Fit Together?

The doctor will put the results of the TNM staging system together to give a picture of the cancer. For example, the doctor might put down the test results as T1 N0 M1. This means that there is a single tumor that is two centimeters across (T1), no evidence of the tumor in the lymph nodes (N0), and evidence that the cancer has spread to other body organs (M1).

Why is Staging Important?

Staging breast cancer using the TNM system is important because it helps the doctor give the right treatment options. If the cancer tumor is deemed to be localized to one area, then local treatment options such as surgery or radiotherapy may be enough to take eradicate it. If the cancer has spread to other parts of the body, local treatment may not be an option, and options such as drug treatments and chemotherapy are considered.

Do Other Forms of Cancer Have Similar Staging Systems?

Yes, they do. Most types of cancer have their form of staging system that is sometimes similar to the TNM staging system. In all cases, the staging systems help doctors describe the magnitude of the tumor, and what treatment options are available for each stage. The other common staging system is the Number System.

The TNM staging system is periodically revised to keep up with advancement in medical technology and treatment. However, such changes are kept to a minimum to allow the system to be relied upon by medical practitioners. A patient's outcome can't be predicted in any way. However, with the TNM staging system, breast cancer malignancy is kept in check, and the data collected helps with the treatment decision.

After Surgery: Taking Care of Yourself

One of the most effective treatment methods for breast cancer is surgery. However, breast surgery requires high technology and specialists. Moreover, postoperative care after breast surgery requires careful steps to avoid any complications. In many cases a patient is released from the hospital with drain tubes after surgery and a set of instructions on how to take care of the wound and what risk factors to avoid. Some helpful information has been compiled below.

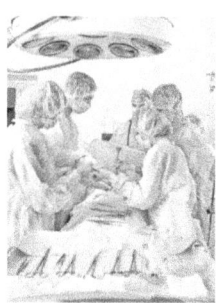

Take Proper Care of Drain Tubes

After surgery a patient will be released with drain tubes attached to the body with an incision near the main surgical wound. The tubes are designed to drain any fluids near the wound and avoid opening up of the wound to drain such fluids. Taking proper care of drain tubes after surgery involves:

a) Ensuring there are no kinks in the tube. This will require you to keep the tubes straight at all times.
b) Empty the bulb when it is 2/3 full or as instructed by a healthcare provider.
c) Clean hands thoroughly before emptying the drain tubes.
d) After emptying the bulb, place it on a flat surface. Flatten it, remove air, and close the stopper.
e) Keep the drain tubes slack to avoid any pain at the incision.

Keep Dry

Keep the wound and the bandages clean and dry. Do not take a shower or go swimming until your doctor allows these activities. Sponge bathing is recommended to stay clean.

DID YOU KNOW?

Drain tubes after surgery are used to drain water, pus, blood, and other body fluids from the wound area. The fluids, if left to accumulate, can lead to infection. The tubes are mainly used in breast surgeries but can also be used in other surgeries such as lymph nodes surgery and even in treatment of fractures such as Bennett's fractures.

Change Bandages Regularly

Change the bandages around the wound once every 24 hours. Ensure the stitches are intact and that there is no excess bleeding. Also observe the coloring of the area surrounding the wound while changing bandages. Any weird coloring like extended redness should be reported to a doctor immediately. For an easy change of the bandages have someone assist you.

Take Prescribed Medications

Take any medications prescribed after the surgery. Make sure you follow all of the instructions for the medications. Sometimes you might require some refills. Some commonly prescribed medicines include painkillers and antibiotics. Avoid any medicine that was not prescribed by your doctor.

Eat a Balanced Diet

Even though your appetite will be off for few days after the surgery make sure to eat. Light foods such as soup are ideal for the first few days. After this period eat a balanced diet with a large amount of fruits and vegetables. Remember you have a wound that needs to heal.

Rest

The quickest way to recovery is to rest. Relax and rest as much as possible. This is the time to sleep as much as possible. Avoid strenuous or stressful activities and situations as much as possible while you still have the drain tubes.

Exercise

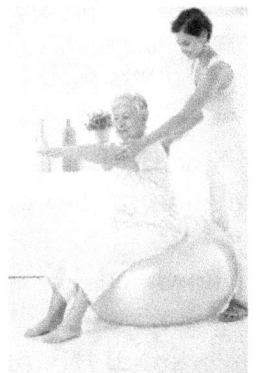

If permitted by your doctor, non-vigorous exercises may help. Walking, for instance, may be ideal for your postoperative care. The hands might be experiencing some tingling and numbness after the surgery and this is the best exercise for them. Be sure to get plenty of fresh air.

Avoid Driving

If taking any pain medications use of machinery or driving should be avoided. Speak to your doctor before resuming these activities even if no longer take the medications.

Attend Follow-Up Appointments

Never miss a follow up appointment after surgery. It does not matter how you are feeling, get some assistance and go for the appointments. Such appointments are vital in detecting anything abnormal such as developing anemia, or infections at the drain site, among others.

Call Your Doctor

Call your doctor if you notice any side effects such as dizziness, severe pain not relieved by medication, heavy bleeding, fever, excessive drainage from the wound, depression, allergies to medication, or a bad odor from the wound.

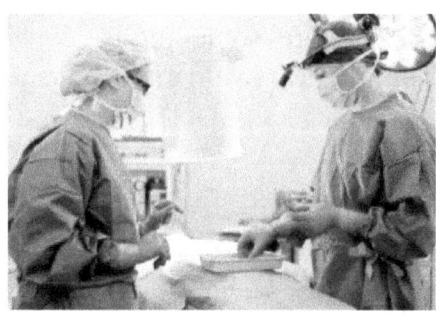

Proper care after any surgery is as important as the surgery itself. Thus the need for careful follow up and postoperative care. Following the above steps will go a long way in ensuring smooth recovery with or without drain tubes. However, doctor's instructions should be followed at all times. Open communication between the doctor and the patient should be encouraged to assist the doctor in detecting any developing issues, including post operative depression or site infection. Moral support coupled with the above steps will lead to quick recovery.

Seven Reasons to Test for A BRCA Mutation

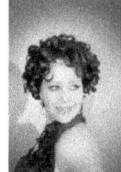

Hereditary breast cancer is relatively uncommon, accounting for approximately 10% of all breast cancer in the United States. Of these women, most will have a mutation in a BRCA gene. Depending on the mutation (BRCA 1 or BRCA 2), the risk for breast cancer is substantially increased (up to 87% lifetime risk) compared to women in the general population (7% lifetime risk.) It is important to identify those women who should be tested for a BRCA mutation so they can be offered more aggressive surveillance and other risk-reduction strategies that can lower their risk of death. Given below are seven indications for testing an individual woman for a BRCA mutation.

1. Personal History of Breast Cancer Before Age 40

Women who are diagnosed with breast cancer before age 40 have an increased risk of carrying a BRCA mutation. BRCA mutations are associated with breast cancer at an early age, most commonly during the premenopausal years. Thus, young women diagnosed with breast cancer should be tested for a BRCA mutation.

2. Personal History of Breast Cancer Before Age 50 in Ashkenazi Jewish Women

Approximately 1% of Ashkenazi Jewish women (predominately from the Middle East and Middle Eastern descent) carry BRCA mutations. Therefore, these women should be tested for BRCA mutations if they are diagnosed with breast cancer before the age of 50.

DID YOU KNOW?

The average cumulative risk for breast cancer in women who test positive for the BRCA 1 mutation is 65% by age 70; however, the risk can be as high as 87% if other risk factors are present that increase the risk further, such as multiple pregnancies.

3. Personal History of Early Breast Cancer and One Relative with Early Breast or Ovarian Cancer

BRCA mutations are also associated with an increased risk for ovarian cancer. A women who is diagnosed with breast cancer before the age of 50 and who has at least one first-degree relative (mother or sister) with a history of breast or ovarian cancer before the age of 50 should also be tested for a BRCA mutation.

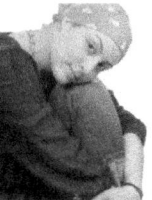

4. Personal and Multiple Family Histories of Breast or Ovarian Cancer at Any Age

A woman with a history of breast cancer who has two or more relatives on the same side of the family with breast or ovarian cancer should be tested for a BRCA mutation. Whereas BRCA mutations result in early onset breast and ovarian cancer in most cases, some families that carry BRCA mutations may have later onset disease. Thus, women with breast cancer who come from families with multiple members on one side who have been diagnosed with breast and/or ovarian cancer should be tested for a BRCA mutation.

5. Personal History of Ovarian Cancer

Any woman at any age, particularly if she is of Ashkenazi Jewish ancestry, who has been diagnosed with ovarian cancer should be tested for a BRCA mutation. Because women with ovarian cancer are often carriers of BRCA mutations, all such women should be tested so that they can be screened more closely for breast cancer.

6. All Men Diagnosed with Breast Cancer

Male breast cancer is very uncommon, accounting for about 1% of all breast cancer diagnosed in the United States. However, men with breast cancer have an increased chance of carrying a BRCA mutation and, thus, they should be tested because, if positive, they can pass the mutation to their offspring.

7. Relatives of Women and Men Who Carry a BRCA Mutation

Relatives of patients who test positive for a BRCA mutation should be offered genetic counseling to see if they are candidates for BRCA screening.

Most cases of breast cancer in the United States occur in postmenopausal women and are not hereditary. In the 10% of patients who have an hereditary form of breast cancer, most women are found to have a mutation in the BRCA gene. Such women typically come from families where there is a high incidence of breast or ovarian cancer, especially in if it is diagnosed in young women or women of Ashkenazi descent. Men with breast cancer also have an increased risk of carrying a BRCA mutation. Understanding who should be tested for a BRCA mutation allows for closer surveillance and other risk-reduction strategies that can lower the risk for death.

What Happens After You Find a Lump?

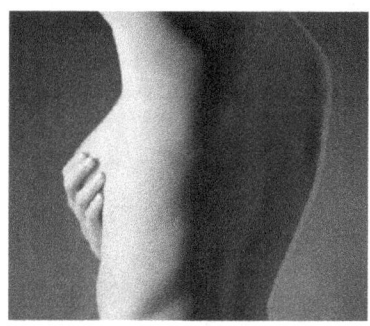

Breasts are made of tissue that varies in texture and consistency. The outer part feels more firm, as opposed to the softer lower parts. This inconsistency has had some women worried that it may be a sign of a cancerous tumor. In most cases the lumpy feeling is nothing to worry about. In other cases, especially if the lump is hard or pronounced, it is time to show concern. If you have found a lump in the breast you should know what to do next.

You Found a Lump. What do you Do?

First of all, don't panic. With the increased awareness of breast cancer finding an unusual lump is bound to cause stress. However, most doctors recommend that you throw panic out of the window, since nine out of 10 lumps are not cancer. It is, however, important to have it checked out. Most lumps will go away on their own, but just to be sure, see a healthcare provider.

It's not Cancer, What can it Be?

Lumps usually form during the menstrual period and will disappear at the end of the cycle. In other cases it could be harmless cysts in the breast. Other times it could be tissue that has just grown past its normal size, which is not cancerous. Regardless, it is important to see the doctor whenever something out of the ordinary appears.

DID YOU KNOW?

Breast cancer is the second to lung cancer in cause of cancer deaths in women. The chances of breast cancer being responsible for a woman's death is about 3 percent, with death rates declining due to earlier detection and increased awareness.

What Should You Look out For?

In some cases, lumps may not be necessary to portend a change in the breasts. Women are thus advised to be breast-aware at all times. In addition to lumps, any signs of thickening, sore spots, discoloration, and overall discomfort should be addressed by the local health provider. If you are unsure about getting checked always err on the side of caution and see the doctor.

The Lump was Examined and Breast Cancer is Suspected. What Next?

If your doctor suspects that the lump may be cancerous, a mammogram and ultrasound should be scheduled to further determine if the lump is indeed a cancerous tumor. A mammogram is similar to x-ray, although it is low dosage. The ultrasound is much safer and gives much more information, such as whether it is a solid or fluid-filled lump. All throughout the screening process, it is important to maintain a positive outlook. Benign tumors are more common than many people think.

What are the Survival Chances for Breast Cancer Patients?

With increased awareness efforts, most types of breast cancer can be detected and treated early, thus helping majority of patients to live long, healthy lives. The trick here is to get mammograms and checkups regularly, so if any abnormal sign of the disease is detected it can be taken care of as soon as possible. Advanced diagnostic equipment and techniques, and better treatment and care facilities have also played a part in the ongoing successful fight against breast cancer.

Can Benign Lumps Increase the Odds of Developing Breast Cancer?

Benign lumps are usually not breast cancer, but some types of lumps that have abnormal cells may increase the odds of developing the disease. A family history of breast cancer increases the odds too, especially in benign lumps cases.

Breast cancer is quickly becoming the foremost form of cancer in the world. While this fact makes it imperative for women to be alert at all times, it is also good to note that lumps form all the time and most are not going to be cancerous. As unsettling as a tumor can be, between 75-87 percent don't result in dire consequences. While it may be harmless, the lump should be checked out to rule out any other complications. Regular self-exams are just as important as a visit to the doctor and shouldn't be ignored.

The Antidepressant Paxil Could Lead to Breast Cancer in Women

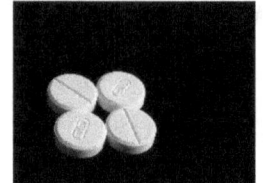

If you are a woman suffering from depression, you may want to speak with your psychiatrist to see if the drugs you are taking are relatively safe and have no known risks for cancer. Taking care of our physical and mental health is very important and those suffering from anxiety, depression, or any other psychological condition should research the risks of the drugs they are taking and discuss any hazards along with benefits of their medication with their doctor(s).

New research from the City of Hope suggests that the antidepressant Paxil has been linked with a weak estrogenic affect that may lead to breast cancer development, according to the Los Angeles Times. This finding is vital to consider, as many breast cancer survivors - as much as 25 percent - are taking anti-depressants due to the toll the disease takes on their psychological well-being. The researchers studied a total of 1,536 compounds to discover which chemicals inhibit aromatase, an enzyme that plays a role in breast cell function.

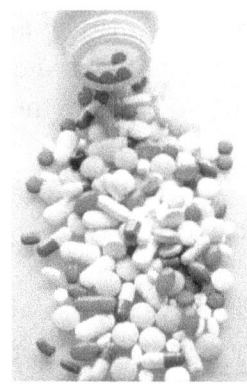

Because many breast cancer survivors have an excess of estrogen already in their system, this extra boost from Paxil could potentially cause cancer recurrence. If you are a survivor, speak to your psychiatrist and oncologist to discuss alternative options to the antidepressant Paxil. This research has also shed light on previous studies where women who were taking both tamoxifen and Paxil had a higher risk of death from breast cancer. It is surmised that Paxil could have prevented a liver enzyme from metabolizing tamoxifen.

"The paroxetine finding helps explain previous studies showing that it reduces tamoxifen therapy's effectiveness," Shiuan Chen, Ph.D., professor and chair of City of Hope's Department of Cancer Biology and lead author of the study, said in a press release. "And it has implications for patients with estrogen-sensitive breast cancer who are on other medications."

This type of information is also important to keep in mind. The way medications mix when in your system could be potentially harmful. Discuss ALL of the medications you are taking with your doctor to see if there could be adverse drug reactions.

Another interesting finding from the research shows that two anti-fungal medications (biconazole and oxyconazole) have a similar effect to medication that is used to prevent breast cancer in women. If you are a breast cancer survivor or the disease runs in your family, please keep these findings in mind and discuss all of the medications you are taking with your physician.

30 Years of Night Shift Work Doubles Risk for Breast Cancer

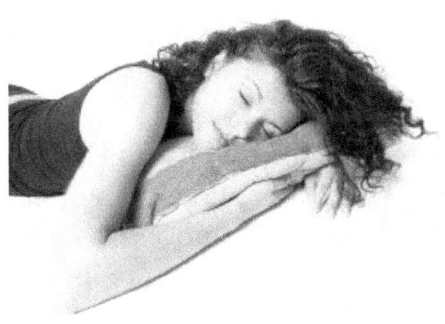

Several studies involving nurses whose careers typically involves shift work have suggested that an irregular work schedule, particularly if the work disrupts normal sleep patterns, may increase the risk for breast cancer. Because other professions such as air traffic controllers and public safety officers often involve shift work, researchers in Canada wanted to investigate the broader association between fluctuating work schedules and the risk for breast cancer.

How many women were involved in the study?

A group of 2313 women in Canada, (Vancouver, British Columbia, and Ontario) whose jobs involved night shift duty were studied to examine the relationship between night shift duty and the risk for breast cancer. Within this group, there were 1134 who were breast cancer survivors and 1179 otherwise healthy women.

What were the results of the study?

Researchers in Canada found that women who worked any type of job that involved night shift work for more than 30 years had a markedly increased risk for breast cancer. Women who worked night shifts for less than 30 years appeared to have no increased risk for breast cancer.

DID YOU KNOW?

Estrogen receptors are proteins that allow estrogen, a hormone made and secreted primarily by the ovaries, to move from the bloodstream into the cells of the breast. Scientists have found that women who work night shifts for more than 30 years have a increased risk for breast cancer tumors that express estrogen receptors.

How much did night shift work increase the risk for breast cancer?

Women who worked night shifts for more than 30 years had twice the risk of breast cancer compared to other women.

What factors might contribute to the increased risk for breast cancer in night shift workers?

Night shift work disrupts the body's normal sleep/wake cycle and the hormones, such as melatonin and glucocorticoids, which regulate this cycle. Researchers have discovered that when melatonin is altered by night shift work, there is a compensatory rise in estrogen levels. Estrogen is a female sex hormone that is known to increase the risk for breast cancer, thus it is hypothesized that the elevation of estrogen observed in night shift workers may contribute to their increased risk for breast cancer.

Women whose jobs involved working night shifts for more than 30 years have twice the risk for breast cancer compared to other women. Night shift work alters the normal sleep/wake cycle and disturbs the hormones, such as melatonin, that control this cycle. When melatonin levels are altered, there is a corresponding elevation in the production of estrogen, which may explain why women who work night shifts for more than 30 years have both an increased risk for breast cancer and an increased risk for tumors that express estrogen receptors.

March 2014

Breast Cancer: Interpreting a Tumor Size Chart

As a woman, you have a 12.5 percent chance of being diagnosed with breast cancer in your lifetime. According to the American Cancer Society, almost 300,000 new cases of breast cancer were diagnosed in 2012. Modern medicine, combined with increased awareness of early warning signs, makes breast cancer a highly curable disease when caught early. How curable depends, in part, on the size of the tumor at the time of diagnosis. Your doctor uses a standardized tumor size chart to determine your prognosis.

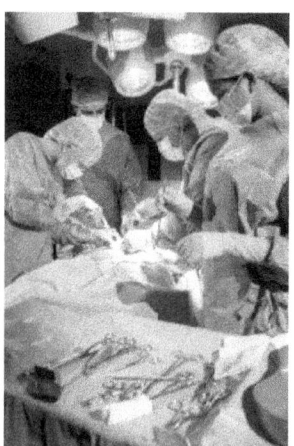

What is a tumor size chart?

A tumor size chart provides your doctor with a reference of how different sizes, stages and types of tumors affect prognosis and treatment. Tumor size is measured in centimeters. Tumor stages are described with Roman numerals. Tumor types are described as in situ, which is also called noninvasive, or as invasive, also known as infiltrating. Tumor types are further broken down based on where in the breast they are located.

How is the size of a tumor measured?

Tumor size is measured in centimeters. One centimeter is a little less than half an inch, or the approximate width of the nail on your pinky finger. On a tumor size chart, tumors are usually represented as circles or spheres, and are captioned with the appropriate centimeter measurement.

EDITOR'S TIP:

If you are looking for some natural remedies for breast cancer tumors, there are a medley of options to consider. Though your cancer is not cured, your immune system is bolstered to help fight the cancerous tissues to a degree. Some of these home treatments include a balanced diet, vitamin D, calcium and the consumption of fruits and vegetables, like broccoli and grapes.

How does a doctor determine the stage of a tumor?

Using the tumor size chart, your doctor determines the tumor size, whether nearby lymph nodes are affected and whether there is metastasis of the tumor. This group of factors determines the stage of the tumor. This type of staging is called TNM staging, for Tumor Size, Nearby Nodes and Metastasis. The stage is then further defined by grouping it into an overall stage, using Roman numerals from 0 to IV, from least serious to most serious.

How do size and stage affect prognosis?

As a very general rule, the smaller a tumor, and the lower the stage, the better the prognosis for five year survival rate. A tumor smaller than 1 centimeter, and in stage 0, I or II offers a 93 percent chance of five year survival. As size and stage increase, five year survival rates decrease.

A tumor size chart is a helpful tool in determining the proper course of treatment as well as prognosis for a breast cancer patient. However, you should keep in mind that cancer treatments and individual responses are highly dependent on a number of factors, such as overall health of the patient and family history. Talk to your doctor about your concerns. Together, you can craft the best outcome for your circumstances.

The Chances of Breast Cancer Metastasizing

Often times, women with breast cancer are curious about statistics regarding metastasis. There are many statistics out there, and they can be frightening. There are many reasons not to even look at them, including the fact that they can be swayed depending on a woman's lifestyle choices. When breast cancer metastasizes, it means that it moves to other areas of a woman's body. With the appropriate resources, a woman can fight her way through breast cancer. Learning more about options can be a great tool to help with this.

The Good News

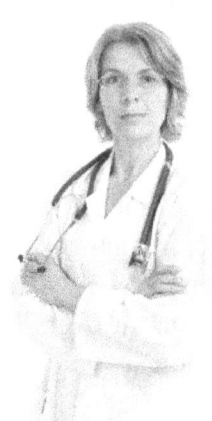

Almost 98 percent of survivors that find breast cancer before it metastasizes, do not have a problem with it metastasizing after 5 years, due to treatment. These are great odds, and can really show how good it is to find breast cancer early, before it spreads anywhere else. There are ways to lower your chances of your breast cancer metastasizing, if you find it early enough. This includes eating healthy, exercising, thinking positive, taking all treatment options available, and perhaps undergoing surgery to remove cancerous cells if your doctor recommends it. Risk factors such as family history can play a part in the chances of breast cancer metastasizing. Doctors use resources to trace the metastasized breast cancer back to other areas of your body. This can be highly beneficial because it means that the cancer is not going undetected. If you have breast cancer that metastasizes, doctors will trace it back to the part of your body where it originated - the breast. From there, both cancers can be treated at the same time.

The Bad News

According to statistics, metastatic breast cancer is going up about 2 percent every single year. Sadly, about 30 percent of women with breast cancer, will find out they have metastatic breast cancer. About 13 percent of these women will not even know that they have breast cancer until it spreads and metastasizes elsewhere. About 2,000 men per year are affected by metastatic breast cancer as well. The breast cancer is found in their breast tissue, and though they are not commonly found to have breast cancer, it is entirely possible. When breast cancer metastasizes, it is about 62 percent less likely to respond successfully to treatment, according to recent statistics. This can vary depending on where it metastasizes. Lymph nodes can be removed, so it makes it a bit easier to treat. The lungs or brain are not easy to treat, and will often be fatal.

EDITOR'S TIP:

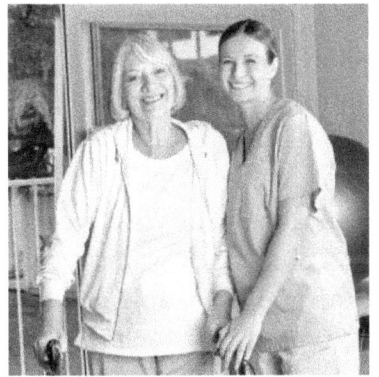

If you are unsure about how to contact resources to help with breast cancer, and possibilities of metastasis, you can talk to your doctor. They will often have information to link you with a support group. From there, you can reach out to other resources that you might find helpful.

Breast cancer is often looked upon as a death sentence, but it's not. If caught early enough, breast cancer may not metastasize, and it will also be more easily treatable. Through routine mammograms and self-breast exams, early detection of breast cancer is better than ever, which brings a better prognosis to patients. Resources that a woman needs include a great support system, a doctor that is willing to fight as hard as she is, and the willpower to keep going. Because breast cancer is becoming more prevalent, knowledge is key.

The Health Benefits of the Thirst-Quenching Watermelon

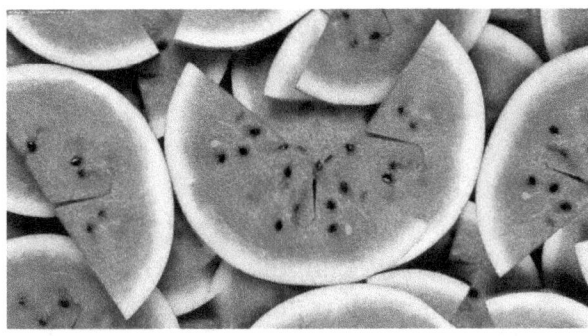

When you have that first bite of a watermelon, the sweet taste bursts in your mouth while the juices start dripping down your chin. You would never have thought that something as sweet as the watermelon could have some significant health benefits and be part of a fresh plant-based diet.

According to Medical News Today, watermelons have plenty of vitamin C, which retains the strength of your immune system, stops cell damage, and keeps teeth healthy. Robust immunity goes a long way to preventing disease such as the common cold or even cancer. This red and green fruit is a good source of vitamin A as well, which boosts eye health. Another interesting vitamin that the watermelon possesses is vitamin B6, which promotes healthy brain function.

The red and juicy parts of the watermelon are full of phytochemicals including lycopene. The substance lycopene can actually protect your body from cellular damage that causes cancer. Additionally, one study found that this fruit can actually prevent some cardiovascular problems such as prehypertension and lower aortic blood pressure.

Watermelon also has an excess of L-citrulline, which has lowered the aches linked to muscle soreness. One study had participants eat watermelon after a difficult exercise session to lower muscle soreness. If you're looking to add potassium to your diet, you 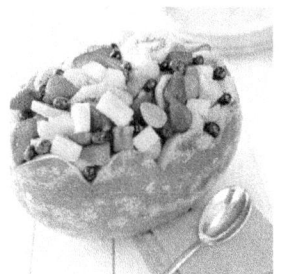 can't go wrong with a slice of watermelon. Potassium will lower high rates of blood pressure and improve muscle and nerve function.

One of the best ways to incorporate watermelon in your weekly diet is to make a fruit salad for dessert. Along with watermelon, some great fruits to add to your salad include pineapple chunks, blueberries, cantaloupe, raspberries, honeydew melon, and strawberries. If you incorporate a plant-based diet into your lifestyle and exercise regularly as well, you will be going a long way toward preventing breast cancer and other diseases.

Breast Lump: Advantages of Early Detection

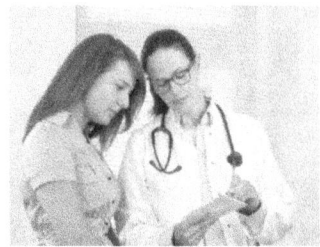 If you feel a lump in your breast, the chances are good that it's a benign cyst. A breast lump that feels like it moves, and is a bit flexible rather than hard and unyielding, is probably a harmless, fluid-filled sac, or cyst. If you have a lump that concerns you, see a doctor. They will perform a clinical breast exam, and might recommend tests to determine the cause of your lump.

What does a Breast Lump Feel Like?

Some women find lumps in their breasts by performing self examinations. Often, these lumps are cysts, which are benign. Cysts are sacs that are full of fluid. When you come across one during a self-exam, it feels slightly rubbery and smooth. When you press on it, it will move a little. When a doctor performs a clinical breast exam, they feel your breasts and the areas under your arms. They palpate these areas carefully to discover any lumps or areas that seem to be out of the ordinary. If they find lumps that don't seem to be benign cysts, they will probably recommend screening tests.

What are Screening Tests?

Screening tests are used to find breast cancer. These include a manual examination of your breasts, and a mammogram. When your doctor examines you, they will feel your breasts and armpits to check for lumps or anything out of the ordinary. A mammogram is an X-ray of your breasts. It can show lumps or areas where cancer might be growing. Magnetic Resonance Imaging (MRI) is being tested in clinical studies for women who are at greater risk of developing breast cancer. Women with a family history of the disease, or who carry a mutated gene known to cause breast cancer, are in this group. Although MRIs have been found to be better at showing breast cancer, they also give abnormal results even when there is no breast cancer.

DID YOU KNOW?

If you've had a breast biopsy, scar tissue might show up on a mammogram as a lump. This can happen with tissue that died following an injury, surgery, or radiation.

When Should You have Screening Tests?

According to the National Cancer Institute, screening mammograms for women under the age of 40 haven't been shown to be helpful. If you're between the ages of 40 and 65, you should talk with your doctor about mammograms. If you received radiation treatments to your chest as a child, for example, as treatment for Hodgkin's disease, you should have regular screening mammograms.

Are There any Risks with Screening Tests?

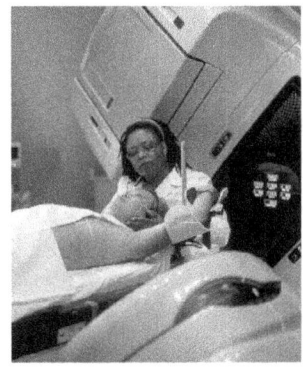

The radiation from mammograms is a very small risk factor for breast cancer, and exposing younger women to the radiation can present a greater risk than not having mammograms. For women over the age of 65, screening tests might have positive results for breast cancer, but these cancers are usually not dangerous. After a positive result, these women might undergo further testing and suffer needless anxiety. Younger women sometimes have false negative results because their breast tissue is dense and tumors are harder to detect. Younger women also have false positive results, along with women who've had breast biopsies, women who have a family history of breast cancer, and women who take hormone-replacement therapy with estrogen and progestin.

A lump in your breast might feel like you can move it around a little. It's smooth and yields to the pressure of your fingers. In these cases, it's probably a cyst, which isn't cancerous. If you have found a breast lump, have your doctor examine it. Ask him or her whether you need to have mammograms on a regular basis to screen for breast cancer.

Get Moving: Physical Activity will Cut Your Breast Cancer Risk

Guess what simple piece of advice was uncovered once again through scientific research and statistical analysis? That's right - exercise reduces breast cancer risk!

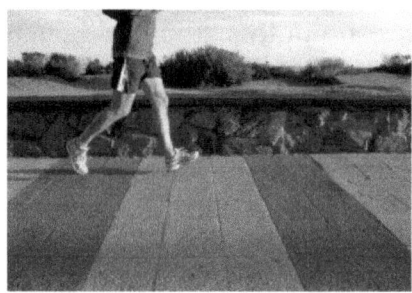

National Public Radio reported that researchers from France analyzed studies following 4 million women around the globe for over 20 years. Women that exercised or were active for more than one hour per day lowered their cancer risk significantly - by at least 12 percent.

Even women who exercised for as little as 15 or 20 minutes a day also saw a reduction in their breast cancer risk. That means moving, swimming, running, dancing, or any other physical activity will improve your overall health.

"This decrease is the same whatever the country, whatever the age, whatever the menopausal status," Mathieu Boniol, research director at the Strathclyde Institute for Global Public Health in Lyon, France, told reporters. "It's very good news."

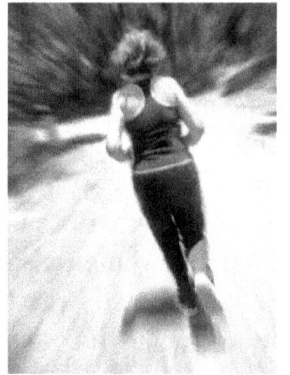

Even postmenopausal women who exercised regularly saw a benefit, as their breast cancer risk also declined. HealthDay News reported that this research found exercise benefited women regardless of their age or body mass index. Additionally, the research suggests that the benefits of exercise are not solely due to weight loss. Along with maintaining a healthy weight, women would keep their breasts healthy by being active.

"These findings are important for all women, irrespective of their age and weight," Dr. Hilary Dobson, chair of the European Breast Cancer Conference's national organizing committee, said in a press release. "Whilst the mechanism for the potentially protective effect of physical activity remains unclear, the analysis, which is presented here, provides women with a real impetus to increase their physical activity by even modest increments."

Along with breast cancer, physical fitness prevents cardiovascular problems and other types of cancers. However, the experts noted that hormone replacement therapy can impede the progress exercise makes. HRT is not wise for women to partake in after the clear indication of its link with breast cancer development. Make sure to exercise, remain at a healthy weight, and avoid HRT in order to prevent breast cancer.

If you're unsure of the best way to start a regular exercise regime, think about your favorite sports from childhood. Additionally, feel free to pick out some fun activities from the list below!

1) Swimming

2) Biking

3) Playing soccer

4) Jogging in your neighborhood

5) Using treadmills at the gym

6) Walking around the block

7) Taking exercise classes like Zumba

8) Signing up for ballroom dancing

9) Ice skating or skiing

10) Flying a kite with your children

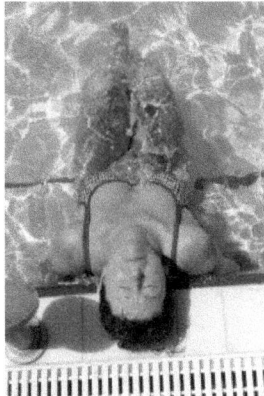

If you partake in physical activities on a regular basis, you will be going a long way toward preventing breast cancer, keeping your heart strong, and living a long and happy life!

April 2014

Peaches Reduce the Risk of Metastatic Breast Cancer in Mice

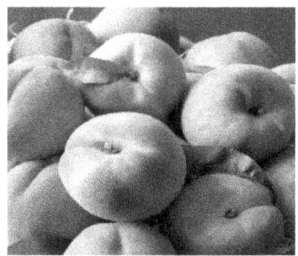
Previous studies have shown that peaches and plums contain phenolic compounds that are capable of killing breast cancer cells. A recent study shows that peaches also reduce the risk of metastatic breast cancer in mice, and may prove useful as a dietary adjuvant in treating women with breast cancer.

Peaches Shown to Reduce the Risk for Metastatic Breast Cancer in Mice

Dr. Luis Cisneros-Zevallos at Texas A&M University has shown previously that the phenolic compounds found in peaches and plums selectively kill breast cancer cells in laboratory experiments. He tested the use of a peach extract in mice prone to a particularly aggressive form of breast cancer that tends to metastasize quickly to the lungs. Dr. Cisneros-Zevallos found that when these mice were given peach extract as part of their diet, the risk for lung metastasis was greatly reduced. In part, this seems to be due to the ability of phenolic compounds to alter gene expression in aggressive breast cancer cells. Dr. Cisneros-Zevallos hopes to translate this discovery to clinical trials involving women with breast cancer.

DID YOU KNOW?

The amount of peach extract Dr. Cisneros-Zevallos used in his study is equivalent to 2-3 peaches a day.

Financial Assistance for Breast Cancer Patients

Breast cancer is one of the most frightening illnesses any woman can have. While modern treatments have greatly increased the possibility of it being cured, it is still emotionally, physically and financially draining. The physical effects of breast cancer can be exacerbated if financial worries create stress. Because of this, many organizations offer free products and services to women suffering from breast cancer.

The Corporate Angel Network

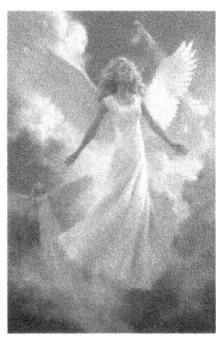

The Corporate Angel Network works with businesses to allow cancer sufferers to access the best treatment for them, wherever it is in the country by arranging for them to fly on corporate jets. The service is open to all cancer sufferers who can walk unassisted and fly without medical attention. To date they have arranged over 40,000 flights. See: The Corporate Angel Network

The Cancer Fund of America

The Cancer Fund of America has a range of basic necessities such as food, clothes and toiletries, which they make available to cancer sufferers from across the country. You need to be enrolled in their program to order online. This can be done by e-mail. See: The Cancer Fund of America

EDITOR'S TIP:

Managing breast cancer has many practical challenges as well as physical and emotional ones. Although being organized may be the last thing on your mind, try to keep your own records of all the treatment you receive. This will enable you to continue to get the best treatment if there are difficulties accessing your medical records (as happened after Hurricane Katrina).

Free Gas USA

Free Gas USA provides free gas to enable breast cancer sufferers to travel to their treatment appointments without having to worry about the cost of getting there and back. The assistance is provided in the form of special cards which can only be used at gas stations. In order to keep their costs down, they request that all applications for assistance be processed online. See: Free Gas USA

Cleaning for a reason

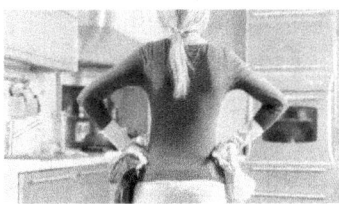

Breast cancer often saps a sufferers energy. Cleaning for a reason partners with cleaning services throughout the country to arrange for sufferers to have their homes professionally cleaned during the course of their illness. They have over 1000 cleaning partners throughout the country. (http://www.cleaningforareason.org).

Breast Friends

Breast Friends provides hats, bras and emotional support to help women with breast cancer feel beautiful again. They also run workshops and retreats for both sufferers and their family and friends. Their support extends to cancer survivors who need help to adjust. See: Breast Friends

Breast cancer is now a beatable illness. Breast cancer sufferers should ideally be able to focus all their energy on fighting for their health rather than battling for their day-to-day needs. By being aware of the free products and services available to them, breast cancer sufferers can ease their financial burden. These organizations are here to help.

Cancer Vaccines: How Far We've Come

We all know how close we are with starting Phase I clinical trials for the first preventive breast cancer vaccine at the Cleveland Clinic. Dr. Vincent Tuohy plans to begin enrolling women in the trials for the vaccine within the next year, according to the Nexstar Broadcasting publication.

"We've known for over 100 years that our immune system can protect us from cancer," Dr. Vincent Tuohy, PhD, immunologist at the Cleveland Clinic, told the source. "These are diseases that we think can be controlled not just by offense, not just by treatment, which is the current paradigm, but by defense."

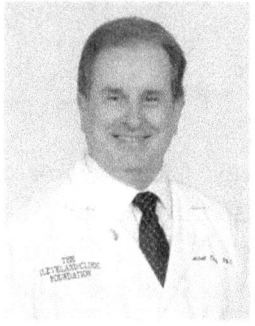

The vaccine works by targeting a substance that is only present in tumor cells and not in healthy cells. If the immune system learns to recognize the harmful entity, the cancer will not grow and the vaccine will, in essence, prevent breast cancer. Tuohy's lab is also working on creating vaccines for ovarian and prostate cancers. The next step is essentially testing the vaccines in humans. The breast cancer vaccine will likely be tested on women at high risk of developing breast cancer to see if it is safe to use. After these initial trials, it will be time to see if the vaccine is effective at preventing breast cancer.

"It's immune software. It's a way of programming your immune system to protect you and keep you healthy," Dr. Tuohy said. "What we want to do is increase our probability. We want to get the head start on these tumors."

HealthDay News reported on another vaccine in the works that may effectively treat melanoma. This vaccine is not preventative but warns the immune system of an early-stage cancer by stimulating dendritic cells that are part of the body's immunity defense.

A different article described the life-saving potential of another vaccine for treating pancreatic cancer. The research followed 90 patients and found that length of life doubled from two therapeutic vaccines.

"Average survival was basically double among those who received the combination compared with the control group," said Stephen Isaacs, CEO of Aduro BioTech, the company that funded the trial. "I think these vaccines may offer hope to patients in what has been a fairly dismal prognosis due to the severity of the disease."

Clearly, vaccines are making headway within cancer research. The new avenue of immunotherapy could have fruitful results in years to come.

Laboratory Study Shows Vitamin A Reverses Breast Cancer Progression

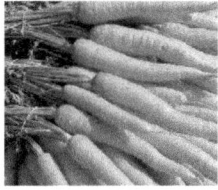

Breast cancer prevention strategies are moving toward identification of dietary factors that can be used to lower the risk for breast cancer. Researchers have found laboratory evidence that vitamin A reverses breast cancer progression. Further studies are needed to determine its clinical efficacy.

Laboratory Evidence That Vitamin A Reverses Breast Cancer Progression

Retinoic acid, a component of vitamin A, was studied in the laboratory of Dr. Sandra Fernandez at Thomas Jefferson University in Philadelphia. Dr. Fernandez exposed four types of breast cells to varying doses of retinoic acid: normal breast cells, pre-cancerous breast cells, breast cancer cells, and highly-aggressive breast cancer cells. She found that when pre-cancerous cells were exposed to a small dose of retinoic acid, they completely reversed to normal breast cells. Even more importantly, the 443 genetic abnormalities recorded in the pre-cancerous cells (compared to the completely normal breast cells) were also reversed after exposure to retinoic acid. Dr. Fernandez hopes to carry her study from the laboratory to the clinic where she can evaluate the use of retinoic acid in lowering the risk for breast cancer in women who do not have the disease but are at an increased risk for it.

DID YOU KNOW?

Sweet potatoes and carrots are particularly high in vitamin A and, thus, retinoic acid. Dr. Fernandez found that a very low dose of retinoic acid was ineffective in reversing pre-cancerous cells to normal breast cells. She also found that higher doses of retinoic acid were less effective in reversing pre-cancerous cells to normal breast cells. She believes that finding just the right dose of retinoic acid will be important once she moves from the laboratory to the clinic. In the meantime, including carrots and sweet potatoes as part of a healthy diet would seem appropriate, and may be beneficial in lowering the risk for breast cancer.

New Study Confirms That Smoking Dramatically Increases the Risk for Breast Cancer

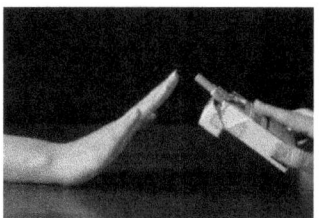

While prior studies examining the relationship between cigarette smoking and breast cancer risk were equivocal and contradictory, recent studies have consistently shown a clear link between the two. The most recent investigation shows a dramatic, 60% increase in breast cancer risk in young smokers.

Does Smoking Increase the Risk for Breast Cancer?

Many older studies examined the possible relationship between cigarette smoking and breast cancer risk. Most of these older studies were poorly designed, and the results were often equivocal or contradictory. However, more recent studies have demonstrated a clear link between smoking and breast cancer. Overall, experts now agree that smoking increases a woman's risk for breast cancer, particularly when a young woman begins smoking during her teens or early twenties.

Seattle Study Reveals That Smoking Dramatically Increases the Risk for Breast Cancer

Dr. Christopher Li of the Fred Hutchinson Cancer Research Center in Seattle, Washington studied a large group of young women (age 20-44) with breast cancer and compared them to a large group of healthy volunteers. He found that women who smoked at least one pack of cigarettes per day for more than ten years had a 60% increased risk for the most common type of breast cancer, called "estrogen-positive" breast cancer. The most aggressive and least common form of breast cancer, called "triple-negative" breast cancer, did not appear to be promoted by cigarette smoking.

DID YOU KNOW?

Cigarette smoking increases the risk for heart disease, stroke, lung cancer, pancreatic cancer, and cervical cancer.

Does pregnancy increase the risk of breast cancer?

Women who have given birth and breast fed their child have a lower incidence of breast cancer.

Can an abortion increase the risk of breast cancer?

There are various studies supporting this theory. One found that if the woman is under 18 or over 35, her chance is increased by up to 800%. That is probably too high, but other studies found abortions increase your risks by 50% or more. Research shows that when a pregnancy is terminated before the milk producing cells have differentiated (which happens at the end of pregnancy), the cells that have rapidly grown in the early part of pregnancy are left in limbo and are susceptible to cancer. This is a very simplified account of the research, but the statistics are just beginning to be accepted by the wider medical community because they are substantial and repeatable.

So can abortion increase breast cancer risk? No, not as far as has been proven. Some pro-life groups have cited inconclusive data to help further their cause, but to date no major cancer organization has made such a claim. Don't take my word for it (In fact, never take anyone's word for it. Do your own investigating.), take the American Cancer Society's word. There's a lot of information to take in on their website, but under "What the Experts Say" you will find: "Induced abortion is not associated with an increase in breast cancer risk." Pretty straightforward, and right from the source.

Does smoking increase rectal cancer risk?

There is a slight increase of risk for rectal cancer in individuals who smoke.

Does breastfeeding increase the risk of breast cancer?

Breastfeeding actually prevents breast cancer.

Do breast implants increase the risk of breast cancer?

There are no studies that demonstrate that breast implants (or other implantable devices) cause cancer. This has been looked at extensively. There was a rat model demonstrating cancer can be caused by implants, however.

Does alcohol consumption and smoking increase your risk of oral cancer?

Yes, alcohol consumption and smoking both greatly increase your risk of oral cancer and combining the two increases the risk even more.

What forms of cancer are commonly found among smokers?

Lung cancer.

What do obesity and alcohol use have in common that increases breast cancer risk?

They increase estrogen levels in the blood.

May 2014

Donating Hair for Those Affected by Breast Cancer

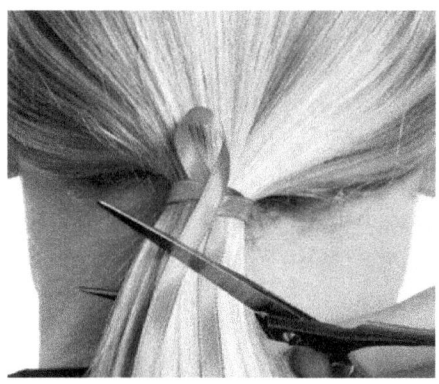

Hair is something people often take for granted until it's gone. While men can find it upsetting to lose hair as part of the aging process, they at least know that some of their peers may be in a similar situation. This is very different to women that have been affected by breast cancer who may feel the loss of their hair as a sign that they are losing their femininity. Cancer wig donations can make a huge difference to women fighting breast cancer.

The American Cancer Society

The American Cancer Society has an informative web page on the physical effects of surviving breast cancer. It features stories from breast cancer survivors so that readers can better understand just how draining and emotionally challenging the recovery process can be and how much it can mean to women to have realistic wigs to replace the hair they have lost. There is also information on organizations which provide help to breast cancer sufferers and survivors trying to improve their appearance and self-esteem. See: The American Cancer Society

TLC

TLC is a non-profit arm of the American Cancer society which is specifically dedicated to helping women suffering from cancer to deal with hair-loss issues. They operate a wig bank, providing free wigs across the United States. They also provide advice on headwear and accessories for cancer sufferers and survivors. See: TLC

EDITOR'S TIP:

The eyes may be the mirror to the soul but your hair is the mirror to your lifestyle. Protein-rich foods are good for hair growth, as is Vitamin B. Hair also benefits from gentle treatment so try to avoid harsh styling tools and products and use bristle brushes rather than nylon ones.

Pantene Beautiful Lengths

Pantene Beautiful Lengths is an initiative run by the Pantene company in partnership with the American Cancer Society, which advises healthy women on how to grow hair long enough and strong enough to be used to make wigs for breast cancer sufferers. It also explains the requirements for donating hair. The site also features personal stories from people involved with the program both as donors and as recipients. (http://www.pantene.com/en-US/pages/index.aspx)

Style Illusions

Style Illusions explains how people use wigs while they are growing back their real hair. It gives readers an insight into the challenges faced by women recovering from breast cancer who want to regrow their own natural hair after it has been destroyed by chemotherapy and how wigs can help. There is also an overview of the different types of wigs available. See: Style Illusions

Organic Color Systems

The Organic Color Systems site is intended for hair-care professionals, but the information can benefit nearly anyone. It goes into detail about how breast cancer treatment can affect hair even after the period of chemotherapy is long finished. The website describes how appropriate hair-care treatments can help mitigate the damage caused by cancer treatments. See: Organic Color Systems

Women who suffer from breast cancer often significantly appreciate the benefit of a quality wig. Although it is possible to buy cheaper wigs made from artificial hair, these simply lack the quality of real-hair wigs. Having a wig made out of real hair can help a breast-cancer sufferer feel feminine again, even if she has lost one or both of her breasts. Cancer wig donation is a small and painless act which can mean the world to a breast cancer victim.

Moving Forward with the Breast Cancer Vaccine

Have you seen breast cancer try to take your life and those around you? Have you feared that your daughter, mother, wife, or sister may be diagnosed with this disease? Wouldn't you do anything you could to prevent breast cancer from taking the lives of your loved ones?

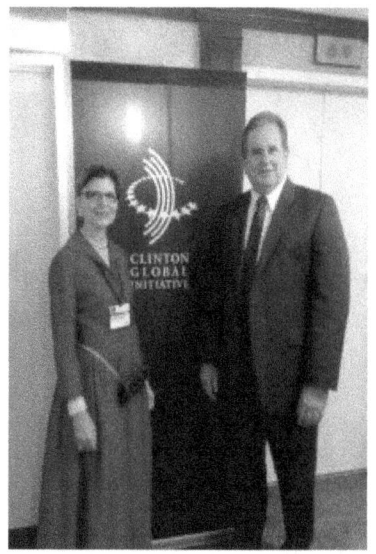

As luck would have it, there might be something in the works right now that could potentially prevent breast cancer in 95 percent of cases. That's right, 95 percent! Dr. Vincent Tuohy of the Cleveland Clinic and his team designed a breast cancer vaccine. The vaccine was found to prevent the disease in 100 percent of the mice tested.

The original research including animal models was published in the Nature Medicine journal in June 2010. Tuohy's team from the Cleveland Clinic's Lerner Research Institute used the compound alpha-lactalbumin as the main property of the breast cancer vaccine. It was found to both prevent tumor formation AND slow down the growth of existing tumors.

Essentially, the study used a control group of mice that were injected with a vaccine without alpha-lactalbumin and an experimental group that was injected with a vaccine containing the relevant compound. All of the mice in the experimental group did not develop breast cancer despite the fact that both groups of mice were genetically predisposed to the disease. The mice in the control group did develop tumors.

"We believe that this vaccine will someday be used to prevent breast cancer in adult women in the same way that vaccines have prevented many childhood diseases," Dr.

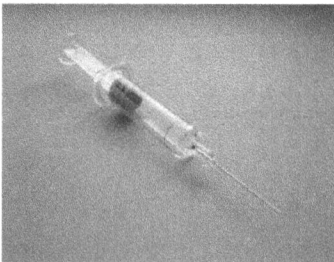

Vincent Tuohy stated in a press release. "If it works in humans the way it works in mice, this will be monumental. We could eliminate breast cancer."

The next steps in this research were clear: find the funding necessary to begin Phase I trials to determine whether the vaccine is safe to use in women. While it was definitely an uphill battle and many common revenue streams for this innovative research declined to help, Dr. Vincent Tuohy was able to gather enough funding to begin the next stage of clinical study at the end of 2013. While the Susan G. Komen Foundation and some other organizations refused funding, there were some smaller grassroots campaigns that helped push forward this research. For instance, Brakes for Breast Cancer, a nonprofit dependent on the proceeds from a handful of auto repair shops, presented Dr. Tuohy with a check for $32,848.84 in February of 2013.

Cleveland Clinic Innovations has created a spin-off company after securing all of the funding called Shield Biotech. The company will continue to improve upon the preventive breast cancer vaccine. Shield Biotech will be finishing preclinical development and seeking FDA permission to begin testing the vaccine as an investigational new drug in human clinical trials.

Phase I clinical trials are expected to begin within the next two years. It will take approximately three years to complete Phase I studies. The Phase IA trial will follow patients with triple-negative breast cancer who have undergone surgery, chemotherapy, and/or radiation treatment.

During this trial, the researchers will be determining the proper dosage and frequency of the vaccine necessary to ensure the highest immune response for preventing breast cancer development.

Phase IB trials will follow the reactions to the vaccine in healthy women who are at high risk for breast cancer and have chosen to undergo bilateral mastectomy to lower their risk. In this trial, the breast tissue specifically will be studied to determine how the vaccine affects the cancer-free cells.

These initial trials are meant to establish the safety of the vaccine and find the best immune response with regard to dosage. Patients will begin enrollment in the trial starting in 2015.

If you hope to help put a stop to breast cancer and ensure future generations of women do not need to suffer through this disease, please support Dr. Vincent Tuohy's research on the first preventive breast cancer vaccine.

Five Foods to Avoid for Better Health

When it comes to preventing cancer and other diseases, we all know about exercise and nutrition. We know to get our daily walks in and to eat plenty of fruits and veggies. But do we know what type of foods to avoid? When we're out in a restaurant, at the mall, or shopping in a grocery store, do we really know what to skip? Below I will outline the type of foods to avoid when out and about.

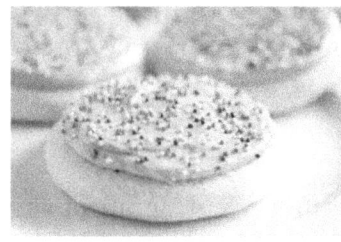

1. Frosting.

If somebody's birthday is coming up and you're planning to bake a cake, consider forgoing the frosting. According to Fitness Magazine, frosting has tons of health risks, as it contains trans fats which raise bad cholesterol and raises inflammation risk. Inflammation could lead to diabetes and heart disease. And, of course, tubes of frosting are full of sugar, which cancer cells thrive on.

2. Processed Baked Goods.

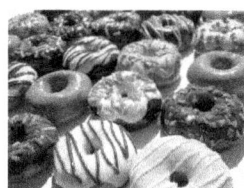

If you think grabbing a donut in the morning is a good idea, think again. Muffins, donuts, pastries, and mini-cakes are not worth ruining our health over. They have too much sugar and worthless calories - and can cause digestion problems as well! The preservatives in these foods are very unhealthy as well. Baked goods like donuts can also cause inflammation of the skin.

3. Soda.

If you only take out one thing on this list from your diet, please make it this one! Soda is one of the worst things for your health! Nutritionists will tell you to get rid of soda from your diet altogether. One can can have as much as 10 packets of sugar in it - drinking Pepsi, Coca Cola, Sprite, etc on a daily basis is a sure-fire way to get diabetes. Instead, try switching to water and fruits. Add some lemon juice to your water to make it more flavorful.

4. Stick Margarine.

Instead of buying margarine in the store, stick to spreading a small amount of butter on your bread instead. Margarine has an excessive amount of trans fats, which will hurt your cholesterol levels. Margarine is also found in certain snack foods, so be sure to check the label!

5. Bacon.

If you have bacon for breakfast, in your salads, or just as a side during dinner, you need to stop this habit! This pork product is high in sodium, fat, and the preservative sodium nitrate. This could cause digestive problems and even cardiovascular concerns. Instead of bacon, add some fruits and nuts to your breakfast cereals or yogurts. Having fruit in the morning could also help you lose extra pounds. Obesity is a big trigger for cancer development and heart problems, so keeping your weight in check is important for your health.

If you avoid the above five foods and cut them out of your diet, you'll be much closer to a healthy lifestyle. Talk to your doctor and see if there is anywhere else your diet could be improved. Make sure to exercise as well. Before you know it, you'll be feeling great and loving life!

Chemo: What to Expect

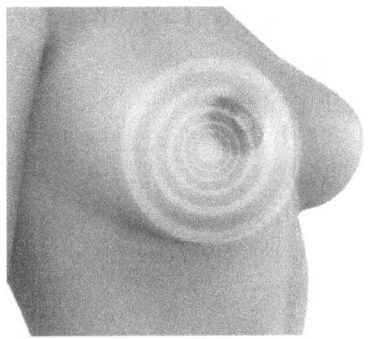

It may surprise a patient to learn that chemotherapy exerts its physical and psychological toll in much the same way as the breast cancer and pain it's meant to treat. The process involves administration of drugs that kill cancerous cells and in the process, healthy cells are affected too. The death of healthy cells during chemotherapy leads to unintended loss of certain body functions and features such as hair or fertility in women. As such, breast cancer patients should know what to expect from chemotherapy in order to prepare psychologically for any result or eventuality.

The Good News

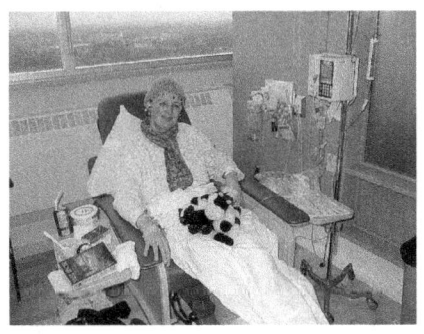

Chemotherapy is a proven medical procedure to treat breast cancer. While the process may kill healthy cells, these have ability to repair and bring back normal body functions. As such, lost hair and other body functions are recoverable. On the other hand, cancer cells are not good at repairing, and this makes chemotherapy appreciably effective. Side effects of chemotherapy are manageable. The process being continuous, other medication or drugs can help ease some of the side effects of chemotherapy. Doctors administering the medication can chip in to help where side effects persist. Unless in isolated cases, the side effects of chemotherapy go away shortly after treatment is completed. Chemotherapy has proven to work well with other therapeutic procedures in the management of breast cancer and pain. For instance, doctors may prescribe certain drugs to reduce the size of the tumor in order to enhance the effectiveness of surgery afterwards. The same may apply after surgery to kill high-grade cancer cells or where the condition has spread to other parts of the body.

The Bad News

Chemotherapy side effects are bad news in their own right. Hair loss, loss of appetite, and diarrhea are some of the treatment discomforts that may feel tougher than breast cancer itself. Chemotherapy may also lead to loss of estrogen and ovary function in women, though some women do recover after treatment. Still, the cancer drugs may reduce immunity of a patient to other infections. Secondly, some chemotherapy side effects are irreversible or long term. Cancer drugs can cause permanent damage to body tissues, organs, or systems. For instance, some women do not regain their fertility after chemotherapy. If the drug causing organ damage is not identified in good time and withdrawn, the results can be permanently devastating. Additionally, chemotherapy may not only fail to treat breast cancer but also cause another cancer. For starters, the need for surgery after chemotherapy stems from the inability of the latter to kill all cancerous cells. What's worse, chemotherapy may expose a cancer survivor to some forms of solid tumors and cancers such as leukemia and lymphomas. The chemotherapy drug used, age of the patient, and other therapies given can raise the risk of secondary cancer.

EDITOR'S TIP:

Keeping records of all the cancers you are treated for or diagnosed with can prove critical to successful treatment for yourself or blood relatives in the future.

When facing treatment for breast cancer and pain, many patients can be highly apprehensive. The apprehension heightens if the patient has to face chemotherapy alongside other medication. However, it is chemotherapy's side effects that scare breast cancer patients the most. The good news is that breast cancer patients can learn to cope with the condition better if armed with information about what transpires before, during, and after chemotherapy.

All about Breast Ultrasounds

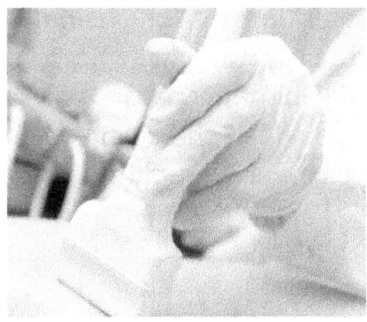

Breast cancer is widely prevalent: One in eight women will be diagnosed with it during their lifetime. Early detection is the key to successful treatment of breast cancer. While mammograms, x-rays, and physical exams are the traditional methods of detecting abnormalities in the breast, scientific advances have led to the use of breast ultrasounds as well. These aid in the identification of any abnormalities, without any negative side effects.

Get an Annual Breast Exam

To detect breast abnormalities, it is highly recommended that you get a breast exam at least once a year. You should also perform a monthly self-exam to detect any changes or lumps between your annual check-ups. It is fairly common for some benign or harmless lumps to be found in the breast. An ultrasound can help determine whether a biopsy of a suspicious lump is warranted.

Determine if You are a Good Candidate for an Ultrasound

A breast ultrasound is recommended for women under age 30 or those with breast implants. This is because younger women have denser breast tissue than older women. This dense tissue is harder for x-rays and mammograms to penetrate, thus increasing the chance of an abnormality being overlooked. Implants, like dense tissue, are harder for x-rays and mammograms to see through. Breast ultrasounds can give a complete picture of the breast in these cases.

DID YOU KNOW?

There are two main types of breast cancer: ductal carcinoma, which occurs in the milk ducts of the breast, and lobular carcinoma, which occurs in the lobules or the areas of the breast that produce milk.

Identify the Type of Lump Found

Ultrasound imaging makes it easier for your doctor to identify the composition of any detected abnormality. A breast ultrasound, for example, can determine if a lump is fluid-filled or solid. One or more fluid-filled lumps or cysts in the breasts are quite common. These cysts are noncancerous and will normally disappear during menopause, unless hormones are being taken. If the lumps are filled with pus, on the other hand, they require draining, followed by an antibiotic treatment. To determine if a solid lump is benign or cancerous, it must be biopsied.

Observe Your Condition over Time

For women who do find an abnormality in the breast, it is vital that they monitor it for any changes over time. In the case of a cyst, while they are usually harmless and require no treatment unless painful, you should still be mindful of any changes in size. As a cyst gets larger, it can become both uncomfortable and painful and may need to be drained. If cancer has been detected, an ultrasound may be able to show if it has spread to other areas of the breast. Results from a breast ultrasound are available after a few days.

With breast cancer affecting women of any age, ultrasounds are effective at detecting masses in the denser breast tissue of young women or those with artificial implants. They detect if any observed lumps are solid or fluid-filled and can aid in observation over time. A breast ultrasound is a non-invasive procedure that can be used during biopsy procedures to help your doctor guide the needle to the area that warrants further investigation.

June 2014

Serious Heart Problems Associated with Chemotherapy

If you were diagnosed with cancer, wouldn't you do all that you can to eradicate the tumor(s) from your body? Wouldn't you want to be cancer-free regardless of the side effects? Isn't it better to have a few side effects than to completely lose your life?

While I may also say yes to these questions and women in this type of situation would likely fight for their life, it is important to understand the risks that go along with some breast cancer treatments. Time Magazine reported that chemotherapy could lead to severe heart problems over time.

The story discusses several cancer patients who beat various stages of breast cancer with the help of chemotherapy. However, in the years following, their cardiologists found that their hearts were not pumping nearly well enough. One woman had a heart pump at 35 percent the normal amount. Today, there is a growing sector called cardio-oncology that is attempting to solve the cardiological problems associated with chemotherapy.

"We're dealing with two devils. We need to balance heart effects with chemo potency, and still get cancer into remission," Dr. Gagan Sahni, director of a cardio-oncology clinic at Mount Sinai in New York, told the source.

Research also shows that few breast cancer patients receive the needed therapy for the heart problems associated with chemotherapy. It is important for any patient taking chemo drugs known to cause heart problems to see a cardiologist before and during their treatment.

Additionally, it is time to develop new strategies in our fight against cancer. It is much better to have treatments that will kill the cancer but will not harm healthy tissues or organs.

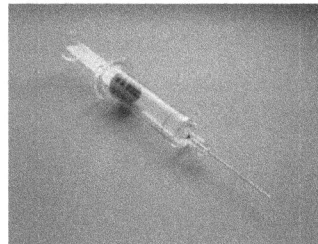

Better yet, the best way to cure breast cancer is to prevent it altogether. Instead of having countless of cancer survivors left with numerous side effects, Cleveland Clinic's preventive breast cancer vaccine could bring us much closer to putting an end to the disease altogether. Please help us spread the word of the vaccine and call on the FDA to approve the start of Phase I trials.

Breast Cancer: The Cost of Taking Arimidex

Hormone therapy is an effective secondary treatment for certain types of breast cancer, such as those that have been identified as being receptive to hormone blockers. After primary treatment, most patients need to remain on hormone therapy for two to five years. The drug Arimidex, generically known as anastrozole, is one of the drugs used in hormone therapy. Many patients are shocked when they discover the cost of the name brand drug and the length of time they need to be on it. However, it is important not to skip hormone therapy, as it the safest best against a recurrence. By preparing ahead of time for Arimidex costs, patients will be better equipped to absorb the cost or find lower priced alternatives.

Benefits

Several studies have shown that Arimidex is more effective than tamoxifen, another popular hormone therapy drug, when used to treat early-stage, hormone-receptor-positive breast cancer in postmenopausal women. Arimidex is shown to increase the time between recurrence in patients who experience this. It shows a reduced risk of cancer spreading to other parts of the body. It also reduces the risk of cancer development in the unaffected breast.

Side Effects

Arimidex is not without its side effects. One of the biggest issues is bone thinning and weakening due to low amounts of estrogen in the body. The drug may also cause bone and joint pain, nausea, vomiting, hot flashes, and fatigue. Many of the common complaints of menopause are also symptoms of taking Arimidex, including weight gain, vaginal dryness, mood changes, difficulty sleeping, and hair and skin changes. Signs of an allergic reaction to Arimidex include chest pain, blurred vision, racing heart, hives, swelling of limbs or head area, and breast pain or new lumps in the breast.

DID YOU KNOW?

According to the World Health Organization, at least 12.6 million people are diagnosed with cancer each year, and that number is steadily rising. More than 7.5 million die of the disease worldwide, and that annual toll is expected to rise to 12 million deaths by the year 2030.

Cost

Arimidex is an expensive, but effective, medication. Arimidex can cost several hundred dollars a month, and not all insurance carriers cover it. At approximately $2,300 a year, most patients will spend over $10,000 to run a five-year course of it. AstraZeneca, the company that makes Arimidex, runs a support network that provides information about prescription programs for patients who are struggling to afford the cost of the medicine.

Alternatives

In 2010, a generic form of Arimidex was approved for sale. Known by the drug name anastrozole, this generic alternative is less than half the cost of brand-name Arimidex. For patients who still need assistance in affording this important medication, many states offer prescription assistance programs. Also, there are numerous nonprofit organizations willing to help.

No matter what the cost, patients prescribed hormone therapy should never skip it. Though there are numerous possible side effects, the benefits of taking Arimidex outweigh them. Once primary cancer treatment is complete, hormone therapy is a patient's only protection against recurrence. There are alternatives to help patients afford this costly drug, even when insurance isn't available or won't cover it.

Nausea After Breast Cancer Surgery: Is It Normal?

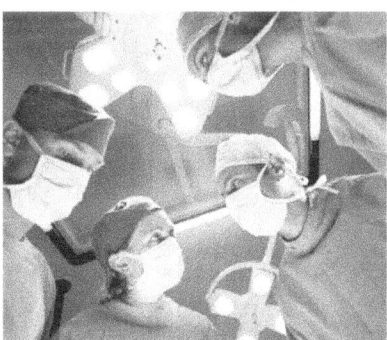

Nausea is a sick feeling in the stomach and is often accompanied by vomiting. If you have received chemotherapy or radiation as part of your breast cancer treatment, you are probably familiar with nauseous feelings. Waking up after breast cancer surgery, you might find yourself overwhelmed by many emotions. You are probably wondering if the operation was successful. If nausea occurs after operation, it is understandable that you are worried. Knowing what to expect and if this is normal will help to ease your mind after surgery.

Preventing Nausea

Well informed anesthesiologists can do a lot to prevent or at least minimize postoperative nausea. One of the possibilities is to give an intravenous preventive medicine before the anesthetic, unless there is a contradiction. Another preventive tactic is motion sickness patch, otherwise used against motion sickness. The patch needs to be applied hours before surgery because it needs time to start working. Other things the anesthesiologist can do to minimize nausea is to administer enough fluids during the operation and to manipulate with different anaesthetics, like using more propofol-based ones.

After the Surgery

In reality, postoperative nausea and vomiting (PONV) are very common in patients who underwent breast cancer surgery. Some believe it is related to the emotional strain the surgery implies and the possible hormonal disruption during the procedure. Nausea is usually caused by the anesthetic drugs used for the purpose of the operation. Patients who had longer operations, such as breast reconstruction, tend to feel sicker afterwards.

Also, nausea shows to be more of a problem with those who received chemotherapy and radiation prior to the surgery. Any nausea should pass within two days.

EDITOR'S TIP:

Even if you do not feel like eating after your surgery because of nauseousness, your body needs food. Especially in the postoperative period you need to supply it with enough nutrients so that you can heal and recover. Some doctors suggest increasing the intake of proteins which are crucial in the healing process. If you can't eat solid foods that contain protein, try protein shakes.

Medication to Relieve Nausea

Anti-sickness drugs called anti-emetics can be given to relieve nausea. They are available in tablet or injection and prove to be effective in most cases. Doctors have an arsenal of anti-emetics to choose from, and they will prescribe a medication that best fits your individual needs. Some of the commonly used PONV medications are metoclopramide, ondansetron, Compazine (prochlorperazine), and even the steroid Decadron (dexamethasone). In recent years, alternative herbal medicine has proven effective in helping to relieve cancer-related nausea.

Helping Yourself

One of the things you can do to relieve nausea is watch what you eat and drink. Pay attention to your body and stay away from foods and even smells that upset your stomach or make you nauseated. It is best to avoid greasy foods all together. Eat several smaller meals per day instead of three big ones. Try ginger tea or other ginger-based products as ginger is known for easing nausea. Another thing you can do is not lay down after eating because this may interrupt the digestive system. Also rinse your mouth after each meal to get rid of bad aftertaste which may trigger the nausea. Besides watching what and how you eat, you could also try acupuncture, which helps some people to manage nausea.

Don't worry if you feel nauseous after your breast cancer surgery. Postoperative nausea and vomiting are very common with this type of surgery. Your doctor will probably prescribe you anti-sickness medication, which will help to relieve your symptoms. You can also take measures yourself, such as eating small portions throughout the day and avoiding foods and smells that make you sick. Nausea should go away within a few days after the surgery. If it doesn't, then it's best to contact your doctor.

Physical Activity Taking a Decline: How to Stay Healthy

Too many people are putting exercise on the back burner. This needs to change! A new study shows that only one in three women who are diagnosed with breast cancer get enough physical fitness according to suggested exercise guidelines. Reuters Health reports that the research used the statistics from the Carolina Breast Cancer Study and was conducted at the Gillings School of Global Public Health at the University of North Carolina at Chapel Hill.

"Physical activity is thought to lower the risk of other diseases among breast cancer survivors, increase their overall quality of life and reduce their mortality from breast cancer and other diseases," Andrew Olshan, who worked on the study, told the news source in an email.

Nearly 2,000 women were studied between the ages of 20 to 74 who were diagnosed with breast cancer within a 3-year time frame. As many as 65 percent of these patients did not meet exercise requirements based on the recommendations of the U.S. Department of Health and Human Services. The organization recommends at least 150 minutes of moderate physical activity per week.

People need to start exercising and moving instead of sitting on the couch all night. There are plenty of ways to get moving. During the warmer months, going for a walk in your neighborhood is a good idea and swimming at your local pool or a nearby lake is also sure to get your activity levels up.

Along with greater exercise, a plant-based diet goes a long way to improving people's health. It is especially important for those battling cancer. Forbes reported that younger women who consume excessive amounts of red meat have a higher chance of being diagnosed with breast cancer.

Frequent red meat consumption can increase your risk by as much as 20 percent. This is why it is so important to continue to eat fruits, vegetables, fish, and poultry. Limiting red meat consumption is important. With a healthy diet and plenty of exercise, you will be at less risk of breast cancer development. So please remember - to stay healthy, keep moving and eat your fruits and veggies!

Breast Health: What to Expect During and After a Surgical Biopsy Procedure

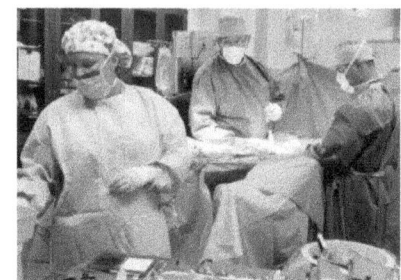

Due to accuracy, many physicians are using a surgical breast biopsy procedure more often than a simple needle biopsy. It is an outpatient procedure and normally requires you to remain in the hospital for only a few hours. Very few complications arise, and those that do are extremely rare.

Why is the doctor performing a surgical breast biopsy procedure?

A surgical breast biopsy has a higher rate of accuracy in detecting breast cancer than a standard needle biopsy. The surgical procedure provides a larger tissue sample of the affected breast mass. This procedure is also known as a partial mastectomy because the entire lump and some healthy tissue may be extracted.

Exactly what happens during a surgical breast biopsy?

Your physician may use mammography, ultrasound or palpitation to locate the mass. You are put to sleep with a general anesthetic. A small incision is made, and some portion of the tumor is removed for testing. After the physician stitches up the incision, the patient goes to recovery.

DID YOU KNOW?

In case the lump is too massive to allow complete removal by surgical biopsy, the doctor performs an incisional breast biopsy, removing a section of the tumor for examination.

How long does it take to recover from a surgical breast biopsy?

Most patients go home the same day of the surgery. Take care of your surgical dressing, and keep it clean and dry. The incision usually leaves a small scar. You can take over-the-counter medications for pain at the surgery site.

Can a surgical breast biopsy procedure lead to serious complications?

Patients rarely develop an infection at the incision site. A scar on the skin and internal breast tissue is visible on future mammograms. Some patients have an allergic reaction to the general anesthesia. These complications are rare and can usually be handled immediately.

The majority of breast lumps turn out to be benign. It is unnecessary to become overly concerned about cancer until your physician receives the biopsy results. You are likely to find out whether the lump is malignant or benign by the time you wake up from general anesthesia.

July 2014

Everything You Should Know About Pegfilgrastim

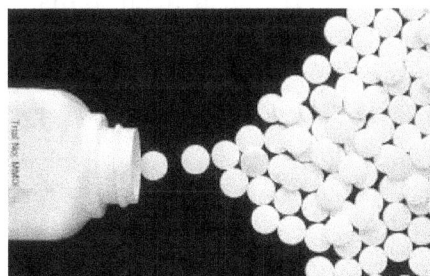

Pegfilgrastim is a medication given through an injection. It is not commonly used, but the purpose of it is to manage illness in folks that are at a high risk for infection. When they are given this shot, it helps their body fight infection harder, to lower their risk of becoming extremely ill. This is given to people with breast cancer, because of the effects that can come from them going through chemotherapy treatments. The cost of this medication will depend on whether or not a person has insurance, and what type.

The Good News

It is possible to give yourself these injections, to avoid a hospital or doctor trip. This can be helpful for some people that like to avoid doctor trips. You will be trained in how to do this, so you feel confident doing it in your home. You can continue a normal diet with this medication. Sometimes with medication that fights illness, people have to remove cheese and yogurt from their diet. With this medication, you do not have to change your diet at all, and can keep eating the same foods you are used to. Some insurance plans will cover this medication. They may require that you go through different treatment before using this medication. Other times they will simply cover it if a doctor orders it. Your specific insurance plan will vary, so speak with a representative from your insurance company.

The Bad News

Pegfilgrastim has side effects. A lot of people report getting a good portion of these side effects, including headache, vomiting, constipation, muscle pain, and more. This medication is extremely expensive, without insurance. On average, a person can expect to pay $3,000 to $7,000 per injection, without insurance. If a person is getting 1 injection every 4-6 weeks, this can be extremely expensive. Pegfilgrastim is said to be about 67 percent effective in fighting infection. This is highly effective according to doctors and past users. It can greatly benefit someone who is at a higher risk of illness.

EDITOR'S TIP:

If you have a problem giving yourself injections, you can speak with your doctor about allowing a nurse to do it for you. In some cases, the doctor may not even let you do it yourself. However, if you feel more comfortable doing it yourself, talk to your doctor.

Breast cancer is a pretty scary thing to go through anyway, but adding the risk of infection or severe illness, and it might even make a person afraid to leave their home. Chemotherapy can weaken the immune system, and this is where Pegfilgrastim comes in. If you find that you can't afford the cost, speak with some low cost clinics in your area. Using this medication to manage white blood cells, and the production of neutrophils is the main purpose, and most people find it beneficial.

Five Foods that Keep Your Breasts Healthy

During the summer, plenty of friends and family have outdoor barbecues to enjoy the sunny afternoons. Often we end up consuming too many hot dogs, burgers, and fried foods during the summer months. A high consumption of red meat can actually increase our risk of cancer. Next time you are at a barbecue get together, consider looking for healthier options. Below we outline a number of foods that will keep your breasts healthy and cancer-free.

1. Carrots and Sweet Potatoes

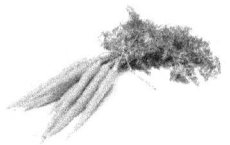
There are a multitude of studies that show carotenoids lead to a reduced risk of breast cancer in women. Foods rich in carotenoids like carrots or sweet potatoes will help manage cell growth, defense, and repair, according to the Huffington Post.

2. Plums and Peaches

Both peaches and plums have a high amount of antioxidants and actually rival the superfood blueberry. In fact, these fruits have polyphenols that can kill breast cancer cells without harming healthy cells. This is truly beneficial when considering that many standard breast cancer treatments like chemotherapy can actually hurt healthy cells.

3. Salmon

One study found that fish oil can actually cut your risk of a common breast cancer called ductal carcinoma. Omega-3 fats in fish oil can reduce inflammation. Researchers recommend women to eat some salmon, sardines, or tuna every week to keep their breasts healthy.

4. Broccoli and brussels sprouts

Cruciferous vegetables like broccoli, kale, or brussels sprouts have a strong phytochemical called sulforaphane that prevents cancer. A study from the Linus Paul Institute shows that this chemical can target and remove cancerous cells while leaving healthy cells unharmed.

5. Tea

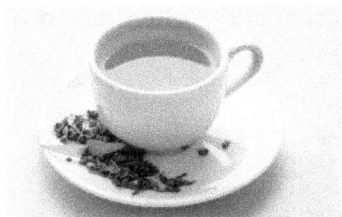

When you wake up in the morning, make yourself a cup of tea. You might also want to brew up some green tea. This drink is full of polyphenols, which are antioxidants that are great for breast health. However, make sure that the tea you do drink is brewed straight from the pot. Often store bought ice tea or the ice teas seen in restaurants have an excess of sugar. Your body does not need extra sugars, as this will only lead to a rise in your obesity risk. For optimal breast health, be sure to brew yourself a morning cup of green tea!

This fine summer, make sure to incorporate these delicious foods in some of your recipes. For dinner tonight, <u>click on this recipe</u> to add two great ingredients known to keep your breasts healthy!

Preparing for Breast Reconstruction after Cancer Surgery

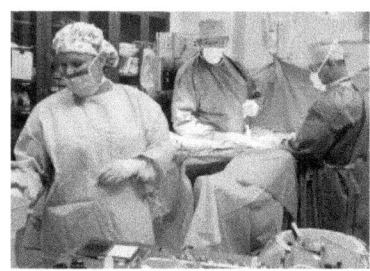

If your breast cancer was discovered early, perhaps you had a segmental mastectomy where only a part of your breast was removed. If your cancer was discovered late in the game, you might have underwent a mastectomy. Afterward, many women choose to undergo breast reconstruction. Today there are many different procedures available for women who underwent breast cancer surgery and want to reconstruct their breast. There are several things you can do while you wait for your operation.

Taking the Time to Heal

It is important that you take the time to heal. A loss of one breast because of cancer brings a big change to your life. As your surgical wounds need time to heal, so do your emotional ones. Give yourself time to adapt to the new situation. Think about why you want breast reconstruction. Is it only to please others or to comply with the image of the ideal woman? Breast reconstruction should be something you do for yourself because you will be the one living with it for the rest of your life. At the same time, be realistic in your expectations. Know that the reconstructed breast will not bring back the one you lost, it will not feel the same as the natural one did, and it might not even look the way you want it to.

Consulting Your Doctor

You should cooperate closely with your doctor in planning the surgery. Before consulting with a doctor, inform yourself so that your questions will be well directed. Make a list of wishes for your new breast and discuss them with your doctor to determine whether they are realistic or not. Don't be afraid to ask questions about anything that worries you. Ask your doctor questions like these:

- For what type of reconstruction am I the best candidate? Will this type of reconstruction fulfill my wishes?

- What can I expect after the surgery?

- What drugs will be used as anaesthetics during the procedure?

- What are the lifetime maintenance requirements for this procedure?

- Will follow-up procedures be necessary?

- What are the risks and the benefits of the procedure?

- What if my other breast won't match the new one?

- A part of the consultation with your doctor should also be talking about the details of the procedure best suited for you.

DID YOU KNOW?

Oftentimes the reconstructed breast does not look like the opposite, remaining breast. The differences can be so big that they cannot be concealed even when covered with a shirt. For this reason, some women decide to have a plastic surgery on their other breast.

With the operation, the breast can be enlarged or reduced in size or lifted to make it look more like the reconstructed breast. Discuss the possibilities with your doctor or surgeon.

Knowing Reconstruction Procedures

There are two main types of breast reconstruction procedures. One is using the expander implant. A tissue expander is a temporary structure placed on the chest wall. Its purpose is to create a soft pocket, which will later contain the implant. In the initial operation, when the structure is placed on the chest wall, the expander is partially filled with saline. After the patient has healed, which normally takes a few weeks, the expansion can be started. The process lasts several months, with the expansion taking place at one, two, or three week intervals. Each time, about the amount of 10 teaspoons of volume is added until the desired volume is reached. Once the expansion has fulfilled its purpose, the second stage of the reconstruction takes place. This will include the tissue expander being changed with the implant and creating a better breast shape. Implants might be a good choice for women who do not have enough of their own tissue to be used for the reconstructed breast, or do not want to have another surgical scar on their body. Another possibility is tissue flaps, where the skin, muscle, fat and blood vessels are taken from the donor site on the patient's body and are then transferred to the breast area. There are different types of tissue flaps, depending on where the tissue is taken from. Flaps can be taken from the upper back, lower abdomen, inner thigh, or even the buttocks. The advantage of the tissue flaps is that they act pretty much the same as the rest of the body and feel more natural.

Getting Ready for Surgery

The doctor will give you a set of specific instructions on what to do prior to the surgery. Requirements will probably include quitting smoking, which vitamins and supplements to take or not to take in the period before the surgery, and instructions about eating and drinking just before the surgery. It is a good idea to make adjustments at home so that you won't need to lift anything heavy in the healing time after the surgery, but still have at hand everything you need. Ask a friend or a family member to give you a ride to the hospital on the day of your surgery and to take you home after you are done.

Breast reconstruction methods were created in an effort to compensate for the removed breast. While not necessary from the medical point of view, they can significantly contribute to your emotional health and help sustain your self-esteem. A decision on which procedure to subdue to should not be rushed. Talk out your concerns with your doctor and inform yourself well about the type of surgery you are considering. Before the operation, observe the instructions given to you by your doctor. By doing all this, you can reduce the stress connected to post-mastectomy breast surgeries and make a decision you are happy with.

Lumpectomy Vs. Mastectomy: The Factors to Consider

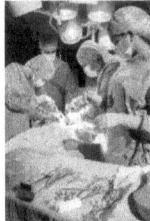 Right now, women around the country are being taught to fear breast cancer and to go to extremes in order to cure the disease. This is being transformed through a higher rate of double and prophylactic mastectomies. In the early 1990s, doctors encouraged women to partake in lumpectomies when their cancer was in the early stages and many took the advice, with the rates of mastectomies decreasing. In today's world, things have changed.

Forbes reported that over the last decade an rise in mastectomies has led to, what some call, an epidemic of breast removal. This may be due to a higher focus on the genetics and family history of breast cancer as well as more trust in reconstructive surgery. However, research has shown that women with stage 1 or stage 2 cancer who remove both breasts do not significantly change their life expectancy when compared to women who choose a lumpectomy. The survival benefit is actually less than 1 percent.

The reasons why some women still choose mastectomies may rely heavily on the fear they feel when they are diagnosed with breast cancer. This is completely understandable. However, the news source explains that many women are actually disappointed by the results after a breast reconstruction. Nonetheless, some women are also concerned with the time and resources required for monitoring the other breast after they are declared cancer-free.

When making the decision of keeping one's breasts or choosing a double mastectomy, women will need to consider all of their options - their current needs and what they wish for the future. One's quality of life after cancer surgery needs to be addressed. Will living with reconstructed breasts be satisfactory? Or will cancer screening more often put your mind at ease? Will you worry about developing cancer in the other breast? Will the financial costs of future treatments cause you emotional stress? All of these factors need to be considered when choosing a mastectomy or a lumpectomy.

Managing Breast Cancer and Metastasis

Metastatic breast cancer, when cancer in the breast spreads to other organs or non-adjacent areas of the body, is a scary thing to deal with. Thanks to the evolution of medical and management techniques, it is something you can live with. Managing the spread of your breast cancer is something you can take into your own hands. The steps below outline one way to manage the spread of your breast cancer and to increase your physical and mental well-being.

Begin Hormone Therapies

Treatment with hormones supplements, such as Arimidex, is one way that you control and manage the spread of your metastatic cancer. Additionally, they have the benefit of fewer side effects as more aggressive treatments such as chemotherapy without sacrificing effectiveness.

Consider Herceptin

Herceptin is an antibody which specifically targets cells that put out too much Her2 protein, something which is present in one quarter of breast cancer cases. A simple application, this can help you manage your condition and generally lengthens life expectancies by over a year alone.

QUOTE:

Metastatic breast cancer may change your life, but it does not prevent you from accomplishing what you set your mind to. One way to manage your cancer is to refuse to let it hold you back and even to use it as motivation to do things you have only dreamt of before. Set new goals for yourself and strive to achieve them, as the distraction and sense of achievement will help you to mentally fortify yourself and to put your life back in your own hands.

Try Chemotherapy

One of the main forms of treating cancers, chemotherapy involves poisoning the body in an attempt to kill or hold off the spread of cancer. For metastatic breast cancer chemotherapy is adjusted to regulate the tumors without hugely affecting the person's lifestyle, and it can provide significant relief and time in spite of some of the sick feelings that are associated with this treatment.

Take Bisphosphonates

Bisphosphonates are a newer class of drugs that come in both pill and injectable forms. These drugs slow down the deterioration of bones and thus can help hold off the type of bone diseases and disorders that might normally afflict those dealing with metastatic breast cancer.

Exercise a Lot

Part of fighting off disease and staying healthy is exercising regularly. It doesn't matter how much you are capable of as long as you get out there and try to work out at least three times a week. The body will strengthen through this process, making your feel better, and the natural endorphins released by exercising should help to hold off the depression that often sets in as a result of a metastatic breast cancer diagnosis.

Monitor Your Diet

Losing weight is a great way to strengthen your body, and your diet in general provides the basic fuel for fighting off disease. People with cancer should generally avoid high calorie foods, such as anything fried, and try to maximize their intake of antioxidants, which help to hold off the spread of cancer by regulating irregular cell growth.

See a Therapist

Metastatic breast cancer is a life changer, and this takes a tough emotional toll on anyone. For many people, personal therapy is a great way to address these issues in confidence and to help yourself deal with all the changes to your life as they arise. While this will not physically fix you, it will mentally stabilize you and, often, that is just as important to managing your cancer and continuing to live your life in spite of it.

Join a Support Group

There are many people who face the same issues as you, and there is no reason you should have to feel alone. Support groups for metastatic breast cancer are available both in urban centers and online. These are a great place to share your worries and experiences with others, and to take in and share strength between one another. Together you all are stronger, and having a safe place to turn where everyone understands what you are going through can be a very comforting experience.

Set New Goals for Yourself

Metastatic breast cancer may change your life, but it does not prevent you from accomplishing what you set your mind to. One way to manage your cancer is to refuse to let it hold you back and even to use it as motivation to do things you have only dreamt of before. Set new goals for yourself and strive to achieve them, as the distraction and sense of achievement will help you to mentally fortify yourself and to put your life back in your own hands.

Learn as Much as You Can

Finally, learn as much as you can about your disease and the treatment and management techniques. Knowledge is power, and the more you know the more you will be able to make the right decisions for your specific situation. This also helps to combat feelings of helplessness that sometimes accompany this form of cancer, and it is an active way to take control of your life again in spite of everything else.

Living with metastatic breast cancer and managing the condition is never easy. It is a trial and a test of your mental fortitude, and you should never be afraid to seek help from others. Remember, though, that your life is not over just because you get the bad news. Try to remain active and set new goals for your life and self in the months and years to come. This way you never forget that you can live your life to the fullest, and that no diagnosis is going to control you, both now and in the years to come.

August 2014

Dr. Ruddy Answers Ten Important Questions

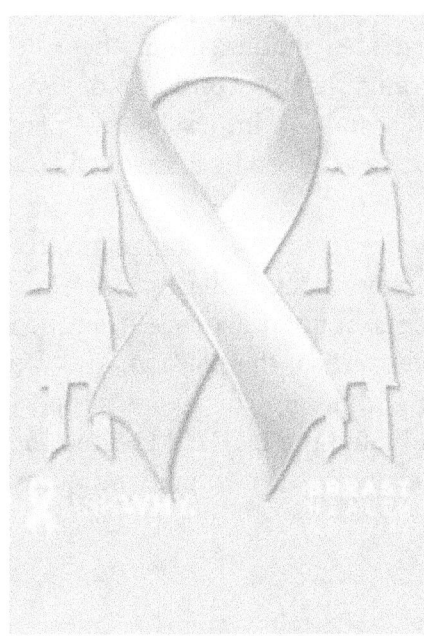

Q: What inspired you to create the Breast Health & Healing Foundation?

A: During the two years I spent traveling the world for the International Masters for Health Leadership (IMHL) at McGillUniversity (2006-08), I underwent a profound metamorphosis in regard to my understanding of how to best address the global burden of breast cancer. Whereas I had been superbly trained at Memorial Sloan-Kettering Cancer Center (1994-95) in the skills and art of breast cancer surgery, and had happily devoted my life to saving as many women as possible from the mutilating and debilitating scourges that attend this disease – a passion that erupted in 1974 when my mother was diagnosed with breast cancer – I came to understand that, try as we might, all in good faith, we could never 'catch up' to this, the "Empress of All Malignancies" simply by racing to find a cure.

Truly, I 'fell off my horse' in the sands of Kuwait, and elsewhere in the world, as I began to appreciate how extensively breast cancer is devastating entire civilizations – old, new, industrialized, agricultural, emerging, developing, or crumbling.

It became abundantly clear that we simply had to understand the causes of breast cancer if we wanted to overcome it; and, therefore, we had to throw at least as much weight into preventing it as we were spending running after it - an increasingly impossible task, given that the incidence of breast cancer had tripled in the decades since my mother was diagnosed!

When I returned to the United States after completing my studies abroad, I approached several of the 'celebrity' breast cancer foundations, appealing to them to open their arms and their pocketbooks to the primary prevention of breast cancer. All they ever did was open their mouths to smile and talk about what a great idea that was, but they did nothing more substantive than to market mammograms as 'prevention', or add 'prevention' to their talking points and slick brochures, or establish impossible-to-meet deadlines for ending the disease – as if breast cancer could be subdued by force of will.

So, I felt that I had to be the change I wanted to see if I was to see any change at all. I looked at all the degrees and certificates and photographs on the walls that line my office; I looked into the plaintive faces of the 6000 patients in my practice; I examined my conscience; and I felt that I had the credentials, the expertise, the passion, and the know-how to throw a shovel for prevention into the dirt and dig up worldwide support for the Pure Cure - prevention. Two months before I graduated the IMHL, I created the Breast Health & Healing Foundation (501c3), and I've devoted myself to cultivating my revolutionary plot ever since.

Q: What is the Pink Virus Project?

A: There is converging and compelling scientific evidence that a virus which causes breast cancer in mice, called the mouse mammary tumor virus (MMTV), may be responsible for 40-75% of human breast cancer. MMTV was discovered by Dr. John Bittner in 1936; it's human equivalent (human mammary tumor virus, HMTV) was discovered by Dr. Beatriz Pogo in 1995. I learned of the existence of this virus in 2006 when Dr. James Holland reported his findings to the annual meeting of the San Antonio Breast Cancer Symposium.

Both of these viruses, MMTV and HMTV, are very similar to HIV, the virus that causes AIDS. By the way, this virus also causes breast cancer in cats. The first thing I did after establishing the Breast Health & Healing Foundation in 2008 was to create the "Pink Virus Project" – my personal quest to raise awareness about the human breast cancer virus. Through this work I hope to support scientists like Pogo and Holland who have committed their professional lives to answering the question that Dr. Bittner first raised almost 100 years ago: "Does a virus cause breast cancer in women?"

Q: How have you spread the word about BHHF's mission to prevent breast cancer?

A: The first thing I did to spread the word about BHHF's mission for the Pure Cure was to create a website and social media links. After creating the "Pink Virus Project" in 2008, I held two Breast Cancer Summits on Capitol Hill. The first was held in 2009 with the help of Senator Susan Collins and the second took place in 2010 with the help of Representative Bill Pascrell.

I created the smart phone app, "Breast Health GPS", which was the #1 breast cancer app in Apple's iTunes store for the first 18 months after its release (2010). I made a short documentary film about the breast cancer virus, "It's Time To Answer The Question", which was nominated Best Film of the Year by Rethink Breast Cancer (2010). I started a blog and have been actively engaged in educating my followers on the Internet about ways they can prevent breast cancer, as well as keeping them up to date with all the exciting developments in breast cancer research.

Additionally, I've written a cookbook, "How to Cook a Revolution", that contains recipes using ingredients that have been shown to reduce the risk for breast cancer. I've become a member of the Harvard School of Public Health's Leadership Council so that I can promote breast cancer prevention throughout the academic community and abroad. With the help of the Harvard School of Public Health and the Loreen Arbus Foundation, I held a third Breast Cancer Summit in New York City in 2013 at which scientists working on the breast cancer virus spoke about their work.

I took that event on the road to the Cambridge Forum in 2013, where it was recorded for National Public Radio. I've become a member of the Clinton Global Initiative, and have used this very dynamic international forum to make the Pink Virus Project the centerpiece of my "Commitment to Action". As part of my Commitment, I am now making a full-length documentary film about the breast cancer virus, "A Pox On Us". I have written a book about the breast cancer virus, and am preparing it now for publication in the fall. Radio interviews, public speaking engagements, and worldwide travel – to Egypt in 2012, by invitation of the University of Michigan's Global Health Initiative – keep me busy and on my toes, sharing my message for the Pure Cure – breast cancer prevention!

Q: What is the most significant outcome regarding breast cancer prevention your organization has played a role in?

A: I think that the most significant outcome produced by the Breast Health & Healing Foundation in spearheading the need for primary prevention of breast cancer worldwide, especially regarding research on the breast cancer virus, is to fundamentally change the conversation about breast cancer. It's what any 'voice in the wilderness' evangelist might hope for: early adoption by other, much bigger players in the field. Although other breast cancer philanthropies initially resisted the need to focus more attention on breast cancer prevention – after all, they are supported and grounded in diagnosis and treatment, for that's "where the money is" – eventually, they had to start talking about causes, prevention, and the virus because, well, I was spreading the word all over Washington, D.C., the Internet, and abroad.

Happily, after that, the Susan G. Komen For The Cure Foundation started to provide some (but no where near enough!) financial support for scientists working on the breast cancer virus; the National Breast Cancer Coalition added the hunt for a breast cancer virus to their "Artemis Project"; and, the Susan Love Foundation included the breast cancer virus and the need for breast cancer prevention on its website. Hurrah, everyone!

All of these things occurred after I created Breast Health & Healing Foundation in April 2008 and began proclaiming the need for the Pure Cure; and the overall emphasis on breast cancer causes and prevention, nationally and internally, has increased ever since.

I'm thrilled with this success, which is really more a matter of imitation by others of the agenda I set six years ago. These organizations have far more power, and much deeper pockets than I; so, that works for me – poor struggling start-up that I still am. But, as Mary Lasker pointed out decades ago, the person who controls the agenda is often the person with the most leverage.

By introducing and insisting that breast cancer prevention, and, especially, research on the breast cancer virus, take center stage in the ring around which the various races are run, I believe that I have made an important, and irrevocable, contribution to ending this disease – sooner, much sooner, I hope, now that everyone is taking prevention more seriously. Of course, I'd like them to take it even more seriously by, say, funding it more seriously rather than just talking about it more earnestly.

Q: What partnerships have you formed during your years as Founder of the Breast Health & Healing Foundation? How have you helped to publicize the world's first preventive breast cancer vaccine developed at the Cleveland Clinic in 2010?

A: Partnerships are key to collective action, the pre-requisite to substantive change. I learned during my studies at McGill University's International Masters for Health Leadership that to be successful, partnerships must be collaborative; that is, each person or organization must be advanced as a result of its relationship to others in the group. That's the secret sauce for change, especially in the current environment where so much is going on everywhere you look – especially in the field of breast cancer! Many of the most important scientists involved in research on the breast cancer virus are now affiliated with the Breast Health & Healing Foundation, as are other international breast cancer experts, scientists, and healthcare leaders.

Certainly, my partnerships with the Harvard School of Public Health and the Clinton Global Initiative have advanced and synergized my vision for the Pure Cure, both nationally and internationally. Having the support of powerful women like Janet Hanson, founder of "85 Broads" (an international group of entrepreneurial women, primarily investment bankers), Professor Nancy Adler (McGillUniversity), Dr. Joyce O'Shaunessey (former Vice President, American Society for Clinical Oncology), and Loreen Arbus (Loreen Arbus Foundation) have added immeasurably to my ability to share my work across a vast spectrum of stakeholders. More importantly, these fabulous women have given me the wonderful opportunity to learn from them about what they do, why they do it, why it's important to them, and how they do it!

My whole-hearted support of Professor Vincent Tuohy of the Cleveland Clinic, the immunologist who developed the world's first preventive breast cancer vaccine in 2010, has been one of the most thrilling commitments of my professional career. Imagine, a preventive breast cancer vaccine. I was shocked and disbelieving at first. Then I read the paper he published in *Nature Medicine* – vetted for more than two years by a panel of experts. Then I called to congratulate him on his discovery, and asked him how I could help support his work.

I invited Dr. Tuohy to join me during the second Breast Cancer Summit I held on Capitol Hill (2011), and at the third Summit held in conjunction with the Harvard School of Public Health in New York City in 2013. My cookbook, "How To Cook A Revolution", is dedicated to Dr. Tuohy and the scientists who are working on the breast cancer virus. Slowly but surely, through blogs, seminars, summits, radio interviews, and personal conversations in Washington, D.C. and around the world, I have been able to explain to a variety of audiences that Dr. Tuohy's preventive breast cancer vaccine is 100% effective in preventing breast cancer in three animal models. I've spread word showing why it is so important to bring the vaccine from the bench into clinical trials to see if it retains both its safety (it's 100% safe in animals) and efficacy (it's 100% effective in animals) in women.

The Cleveland Clinic has taken the lead in promoting Dr. Tuohy's vaccine: it has made the vaccine, which I call the "Pink Vaccine" – and, now, it does likewise - the centerpiece of its fundraising campaign. I'm happy to report that last year the Cleveland Clinic spun off a private entity (Shield Biotech) to fund clinical trials to test the vaccine in women. The week after this was announced in September 2013, I invited Dr. Tuohy to address a group of attendees at the annual meeting of the Clinton Global Initiative in New York City, and then I invited him to address the audience during my presentation to the Cambridge Forum in Boston, October 2013.

I'm not sure where our next 'joint venture' will take place, but I'm looking forward to his clinical trials, and I await the results of testing his vaccine in women with hopeful, bated breath. I will keep an open mind, and a skeptical view to the outcome. As Dr. Larry Norton of Memorial Sloan-Kettering said of Tuohy's vaccine in 2010, when it first appeared in *Nature Medicine:* "Not everything that works in mice, works in women." Indeed, that is true. I know Dr. Norton. I've worked with him. He is wonderful and brilliant. But, let me add: Everything that now works in women, first worked in mice. Let's see if this one does too.

Q: What type of projects or events have you put on to spread awareness about breast cancer prevention?

A: The three Breast Cancer Summits (two in Washington, D.C, and one in New York City) have been the hallmark events to spread the word about breast cancer prevention. I made an app for the iPad, "Breast Cancer 411" that includes all the known and proven ways that women can reduce their risk for breast cancer. All my apps are free, so they have received broad uptake around the world.

The short documentary film about the breast cancer virus I made in 2010, "It's Time To Answer The Question" has received over 5000 views on You Tube – not as much as the cat playing the piano, but it's a start. I expect that the full documentary film, "A Pox On Us", which will be submitted to film festivals worldwide (2015), will gain greater traction. The proceeds from the sale and distribution of the film will be used to fund the first international breast cancer conference for the breast cancer virus.

I think that getting all the scientists who are working on the virus in one room for three days, and in front of other scientists who are familiar with viruses and cancer and vaccines, would be a real game-changer among the academic community. From there I expect it will spill out of the ivory towers and down into the streets of mainstream medicine. I'm really looking forward to this event as the next big step for Breast Health & Healing.

I also expect that when my book about the breast cancer virus comes out in the fall, the tipping point for the Pure Cure will settle precisely into the crosshairs of breast cancer awareness. I feel certain that when women learn about the virus, and understand the importance of this research, they will rise up with one voice and demand that enough money be given to support these scientists so that their work can be completed, at last. My blogs, and constant talking about breast cancer prevention, the virus, and the vaccine continue to spread awareness for the Pure Cure. So much so, that if you do a Google search for 'breast cancer virus', and click on "images", you will see a photograph of me – a viral messenger, of sort, for breast cancer prevention.

Q: What has been the most surprising thing about running your own non-profit foundation?

A: The most surprising thing I discovered about running a non-profit foundation is how difficult it is to raise money. Yikes! Especially for me – double yikes! I was raised with the understanding that if you wanted or needed money, then you went out and earned it, which is what I always did.

My first job, selling shoes. My second job, waiting the soda fountain at the Woolworth's in Augusta, Georgia. (Twenty-five cent tips made my day, circa 1969.) The idea of asking people for money, even for a worthy cause, seems so foreign to me that I have no skills – or stomach – for it. So, I have settled into my limitations, and have simply funded the foundation with my own income.

Occasionally, I will receive donations from grateful patients or local merchants who want to help support the Pure Cure. And I'm always deeply grateful to them for that. But I have discovered that I am more suited to teaching than to fundraising; and, so, I stick to doing that. I'm happy to fund the work of the Breast Health & Healing Foundation, largely alone, for I really believe I am called to do it.

Besides, do I really want to sell my logo to make money if it means slapping it on, say, buckets of fried chicken, or plastering it on every pink plastic thing in sight? No. In the spirit of earning rather than asking for help – how I was raised - I hope that when my book comes out, its sales will generate enough money for the Breast Health & Healing Foundation to empower my work even further.

There was another, as surprising but more disturbing, discovery that I made soon after I created the Breast Health & Healing Foundation: The competition among breast cancer foundations is as fierce as anything to be found on the Serengetti. The behavior of many (but, not all) of these organizations is nothing short of ruthless! I was shocked. Perhaps I had been in medicine too long, and had grown up believing in the humanity and generosity of philanthropy. But, boy, breast cancer philanthropy is a business as serious as selling stocks! Look to Wall Street to understand the rules. Beware the wolves that run the show.

I decided very early on that I'd rather not play rugby with these people. Instead, I have chosen to work on the periphery, as best I can, with pen and blog and microphone, to coach the scrum in the direction of the causes and prevention of breast cancer. When I finally see them cross the goal, with a virus or vaccine in hand, I will stand up in my bleacher and cheer their victory, satisfied they've put points on the board for the Pure Cure.

The Best Types of Wigs for Cancer Victims

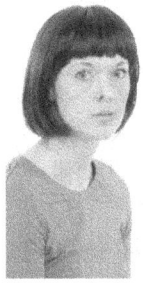 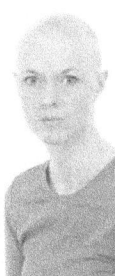

One of the side effects of chemotherapy is hair loss. Why does hair loss occur during chemotherapy and radiation? Hair consists of cells that are fast growing, and cancer cells also tend to grow quickly, making them similar types of cells. Chemotherapy and radiation therapy are designed to eliminate all cells that are fast-growing in nature, so hair cells are targeted by the treatment just like cancer cells are. Most hair loss is temporary, however, and depends on the length and strength of the treatments. Some people lose a little hair, though others lose all of their hair during cancer treatments. While some people choose to wrap their heads in a scarf, some do nothing and others choose chemo wigs. The goals in choosing a chemo wig are to choose one that looks natural and to choose one that fits well. With that in mind, what are the options for wigs for people who are undergoing cancer treatments?

The Good News

Human hair or synthetic hair wigs are the two choices of wig types. Synthetic hair is easier to take care of and is less costly, while synthetic wigs dry faster than real human hair wigs do, making them a time-saver. The lower cost and ease of care and maintenance makes synthetic chemo wigs a more appealing option for many cancer patients with hair loss as well. Human hair feels more like real hair does, which makes wigs that are made from it appealing to some people who have the money and time for one. Human hair wigs can also be styled in various ways. Other types of chemo wigs include machine-made, hand-sewn or custom wigs. Wigs can be purchased online, but it is usually better to try them on to test the fit, the style and the comfort of the wig. There are specialists that deal in wigs for patients who are undergoing chemo and radiation, and some insurance providers have special coverage for cancer patients that covers wigs and wig consultations.

The Bad News

Real human hair wigs can come with a starting price tag of $1,000 and require more care and maintenance than synthetic hair does. Synthetic wigs come in one style and that cannot usually be changed. Once it has been set by the manufacturer, even washing it will not change the style. A person undergoing cancer treatments that feels well enough, has the finances, has the time and wants to style a human hair wig will often find this type of wig appealing. Otherwise, the synthetic type is a better solution. All chemo wigs, regardless of type, style and attributes, have to be washed and set at least once a week if they are worn on a regular basis. If the person using a human hair wig does not have experience with the care and maintenance of these wigs, then professional services are a good course of action. This will ensure that the wig is well maintained and looks good, because human hair requires more special care for washing and styling than synthetic hair wigs do.

EDITOR'S TIP:

It is important to choose a wig that fits your personal style, because that type of consideration is crucial to how you feel about yourself and to how you look.

Comfort is important when choosing a wig. If the wig feels uncomfortable or does not fit well, then it is not as functional as it needs to be for the patient. The best type of wig for a cancer patient is one that fits, one that is comfortable and functional, one that is easy to maintain and one that makes them feel good about themselves in an otherwise stressful situation. The ideal wig for an individual is one that is affordable for them and that makes them happy.

Breast Cancer Genetics Explodes - Third Gene Identified as a Cause

Cancer research has uncovered a huge discovery for women everywhere. A new gene mutation called PALB2 has just as much risk for breast cancer development as the BRCA1 and BRCA2 mutations, the New York Times reported.

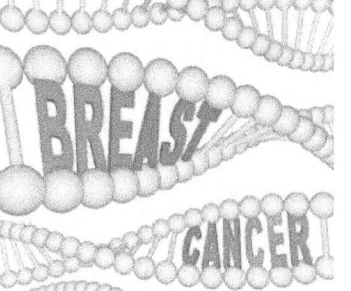

Researchers from the University of Cambridge studied 362 subjects with PALB2 mutations who did not have the same defect in their BRCA genes. However, all of these patients had at least one family member with breast cancer. Out of all subjects, 311 women and 51 men had PALB2 mutations. From those numbers, 229 women and 7 men were diagnosed with breast cancer.

This research can be found in The New England Journal of Medicine. The statistics show that carriers of this genetic defect have a 35 percent chance of developing breast cancer by age 70. It was also found that younger women with the genetic mutation were at higher risk of the disease. Another interesting finding is that women with the PALB2 mutation were at higher risk of triple-negative breast cancer, which is more aggressive than other types.

"This has to be tailored to the patients, who may have other mutations and varying family risk," Dr. Anees B. Chagpar, the director of the breast center at Yale-New Haven Hospital, told the source. "With no family history, the increase they found is 35 percent. If you have two or more family members with cancer, they found a risk of 58 percent."

The research comes from patients around the world - eight separate countries and 14 sites were used to screen for the genetic defect. The researchers suggest that women who have a family history of breast cancer and are negative for BRCA1/2 gene mutations to test for PALB2.

"It is by far the largest study to date and provides the most accurate risk estimates for PALB2 mutation carriers," study co-author Dr. Marc Tischkowitz told Healthline. "It shows that the breast cancer risk is modified by family history."

Along with the BRCA genes, doctors and patients alike will now need to pay attention to the risks associated with PALB2 gene mutations.

Sudden Signs of Breast Cancer

The truth about breast cancer or about any type of breast growth is that few symptoms develop in the early stages. Sometimes, a breast growth is found during a routine exam or after a mammogram and many women are shocked because they don't feel sick. Seldom are there any sudden signs of breast cancer, though there are some signs that some women may not be aware of when it comes to breast cancer. Here is some information that you need to know regarding breast health.

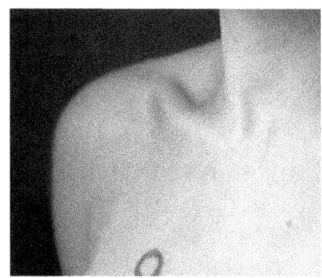

The Good News

Women are told from an early age to be aware of breast lumps or of any other changes that might occur in their breasts. Breast lumps are not necessarily the first sign of cancer, and in fact, breast lumps are fairly common and are usually not cancerous in most cases. Breast cancer symptoms can vary depending on several factors. Some of these factors can include the size of the growth, the position of the growth, the location of the growth and the type of growth.

It is uncommon for pain to be a sign of breast cancer, but it can be one of the symptoms in certain types of malignant tumors. Even when a cancerous tumor is discovered upon a routine exam or due to breast pain, most cases are easily diagnosed and are successfully treated. Due to better cancer screening methods and awareness of breast cancer, it is caught early enough to save lives most of the time. The survival rates for breast cancer are very high, and they vary depending on the type of cancer, as well as the nature of the cancer.

The Bad News

There are certain signs of breast cancer with which every woman should be familiar. These are the less common signs that are crucial to know, and they can include:

- Soreness, itchiness or redness of the breast(s)

- Upper back pain (between the shoulder blades)

- Nipple changes from a tumor growing just under the nipple

- Changes in the size or shape of a breast

- Swelling, pain or a lump discovered in your armpit.

These symptoms can all be accompanied by breast pain, or there may be no pain at all in the breasts. Due to the location of certain breast cancers, it can spread to the lymph nodes and to other parts of the body including the lungs, the bones and the brain. How the cancer spreads (or metastasizes) depends on the type of cancer being treated as well as how long it has been neglected.

The most common signs of breast cancer can include a thickening of breast tissue or a lump, bloody discharge coming from the nipple, dimpling of the breast or other skin changes on the breast, an inverted nipple, flaking or scaling of the breast skin or on the nipple and/or pitting of the breast skin that can resemble that of an orange's skin.

EDITOR'S TIP:

You should not ignore any changes in your breasts even if you have just had a mammogram and it came back clear. Report these changes to your doctor and let him or her determine the best course of action.

Even with the knowledge that most breast lumps are not cancerous, it is still very important to get checked any time that there are changes in the breasts. Sudden weight loss or sudden weight gain, unexplained pains in the breasts or back and any kind of change in how your breasts or nipples look or feel need to be immediately addressed with your doctor. You cannot take chances with breast cancer, or with any kind of cancer for that matter. It is vital that you take charge of your health care by being informed and by taking action when you notice even a minor change in your breasts.

Tamoxifen Reduces the Risk of Contralateral Breast Cancer in Survivors with BRCA Mutations

Women who carry BRCA 1 or 2 mutations have the highest risk for breast cancer, as much as 85% over the course of their lifetime. At the present time, the most effective way to reduce that risk is to have bilateral prophylactic mastectomy along with removal of the ovaries. The use of other prevention strategies, such as drug therapy with anti-estrogens like tamoxifen that are known to reduce the risk for breast cancer, has long been sought as a way for BRCA carriers to avoid mutilating and often debilitating surgery. Scientists in Australia have just published an article showing that tamoxifen therapy can reduce the risk of breast cancer in BRCA carriers by as much as 58%.

Who conducted the study of tamoxifen therapy in BRCA carriers?

Dr. Kelly-Anne Phillips of the University of Melbourne in Australia conducted a study of BRCA carriers who had been diagnosed with breast cancer and were then placed on tamoxifen therapy.

What were the details of the study?

Dr. Phillips studied 1583 women with a BRCA 1 mutation and 881 women with a BRCA 2 mutation who had been diagnosed with cancer in one breast (after 1970) and who had subsequently been placed on the anti-estrogen drug tamoxifen, which blocks the growth and spread of tumors that are sensitive to estrogen.

DID YOU KNOW?

Only 1 in 5 women in Australia who carry a BRCA mutation elect to have bilateral prophylactic mastectomy to reduce their lifetime risk for breast cancer.

What were the results of the study?

Dr. Phillips found that 24% of the 1583 women with a BRCA 1 mutation and 52% of the 881 women with a BRCA 2 mutation had been given tamoxifen as part of their treatment for breast cancer. Tamoxifen proved to be very beneficial in preventing breast cancer recurrence in the opposite breast, known as contralateral breast cancer (CBC). Women with a BRCA 1 mutation who took tamoxifen had a 58% reduction in the incidence of CBC; women with a BRCA 2 mutation had a 48% reduction in CBC.

What were the conclusions of the study?

Tamoxifen was found to reduce the risk for CBC in women with BRCA mutations by approximately 50% overall.

Tamoxifen is an anti-estrogen drug that reduces the risk for breast cancer by blocking the growth-stimulating effects of estrogen on the majority of breast cancer tumors. Women with BRCA mutations have the highest risk for breast cancer, as much as 85% over the course of their lifetime. Bilateral prophylactic mastectomy and removal of the ovaries has been the primary prevention strategy to reduce the risk for breast cancer in BRCA mutation carriers, but a recent study conducted at the University of Melbourne in Australia now demonstrates that tamoxifen therapy can reduce the risk for contralateral breast cancer in BRCA mutation survivors, on average, 50%.

September 2014

The Pink Virus Documentary: Our Story Needs to be Told

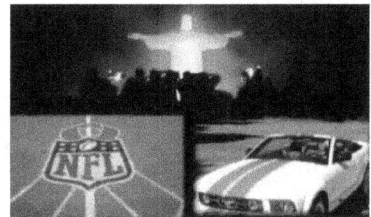

October or National Breast Cancer Awareness Month is one week away. This month has led companies around the country to dye their products pink and sell merchandise in an effort to raise money for breast cancer research, treatments, and care. However, the money that may be donated to the largest breast cancer charities are not always spent the way we may think. For example. out of all the funding that the Susan G. Komen Foundation receives, only between 15.5 percent to 26 percent of it goes to breast cancer research grants, according to the Chronicle of Philanthropy. To check out Komen's 2012 financial data report, click here.

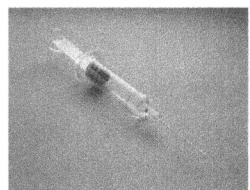

Most importantly, breast cancer prevention - specifically the research behind the breast cancer virus and vaccine - seems to get left behind in the dust. Less than 2 percent of all breast cancer funding goes to prevention despite the fact that hundreds of millions of grants exist to target this disease every year.

If we are going to change the way nonprofits work and the healthcare system runs, we will need to transform our ways of thinking. Breast cancer has become a disease to treat instead of prevent due to the millions of dollars it pumps into the healthcare and pharmaceutical sector every year. Do we want to save women's lives or support the economy? It is time for a change.

We need to answer two important questions in order to get the ball rolling. These questions are:

1. Does a virus cause breast cancer in women?

2. Can we make a safe and effective vaccine that prevents breast cancer in women?

The Breast Health and Healing Foundation has partnered with Soapbox Entertainment and They Say We Are Dreamers to start the development of an incredible documentary film about the breast cancer virus and vaccine. The film is called "The Pink Virus: A Pox on Us." It details the discovery of the mouse mammary tumor virus, which could be responsible for a large amount of human breast cancers, as well as Cleveland Clinic's first preventive breast cancer vaccine known to keep 100 percent of tested mice from developing the disease.

This research needs to be shared. Further funding needs to be gathered and we need to revolutionize the whole concept of treating disease and emphasize prevention. This documentary film needs to be finished so we can finally tell our story around the nation. However, we refuse to ask for help from corporate sponsors on this project. This will be different from the pink merchandise you see around the stores every October.

As such, we need your help! We are looking to crowd-fund in order to complete this documentary film. We will gather the funds $20 at a time, $30 at a time, but we will gain the money we need to tell our story. We need your help. Whether you can help by donating or by sharing the information with your family and friends, please do so. This story needs to be told. Only you can help us tell it.

Donate here to the Pink Virus documentary film!

Breast Healthy Recipe: Roasted Brussels Sprouts

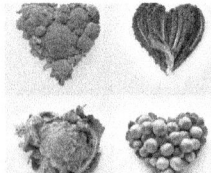

Dr. Dorothy Pathak, an epidemiologist trained at Harvard University who now works at Michigan State University, discovered that Polish immigrants living in Chicago and Detroit had three times the risk for breast cancer compared with their countrymen back home. After studying the possible reasons for the dramatic increase in breast cancer risk in these newly Americanized women, Pathak discovered that cabbage was at the heart of the problem - or more precisely, lack of cabbage. When the Polish women immigrated to the United States, they gave up eating cabbage with the same regularity as they had done back home. Pathak found that by returning cabbage to the diet three times a week the risk for breast cancer returned to the lower levels found in Poland. Scientists now know that cabbage, a cruciferous vegetable, contains nutrients that block cancer activity in many tumors, especially breast and prostate cancer.

Brussels sprouts are members of the cabbage family, and although they can be bitter if eaten raw, once they're roasted they take on a sweetly delicate flavor. They pair exceptionally well with roasted meats.

PREP TIME: 10 minutes

COOK TIME: 30 minutes

READY IN: 40 minutes

Ingredients

24 - brussels sprouts

1/4 - extra virgin olive oil

Directions

Preheat oven to 400 degrees. Wash the brussels sprouts, remove the outer leaves if soiled, and cut them in half. Place the brussels sprouts into a large bowl and toss them with the olive oil. Place the brussels sprouts, cut side down, on a large baking sheet. Roast for 15 minutes. Turn them over on the baking sheet and roast for another 15 minutes. Remove from the oven and sprinkle with salt and pepper to taste.

The brussels sprouts can be reheated in the microwave, and thus make an excellent vegetable to take to work for lunch or reheat for dinner on another night.

Cabbage is an inexpensive vegetable, very cost-effective pound for pound. It provides vitamins and loads of fiber, and it appears to lower the risk for breast cancer in women who eat it at least three times a week.

DID YOU KNOW?

Scientists exposed cancer cells to extracts of cabbage (in amounts that a normal person would consume in a daily diet that included cabbage.) The cancer cells stopped growing.

Exercise Your Way to Breast Cancer Prevention

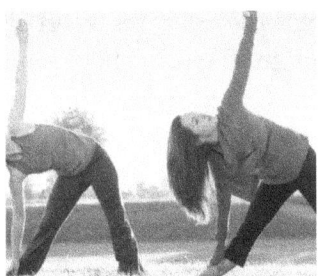

Several large epidemiologic studies have shown that regular exercise lowers the risk for breast cancer. But how much exercise, and how often, and does it work for older as well as younger women? These are some of the open questions that remain to be answered. However a recent investigation conducted by the University of North Carolina School of Global Public Health addressed these questions and clarified some of the subtleties concerning exercise as breast cancer preventative.

How many women were involved in the University of North Carolina study?

There were 1504 women with breast cancer (233 with non-invasive breast cancer and 1271 with invasive breast cancer) and 1555 healthy women involved in the study.

What were the ages of the women in the study?

Women in the study were 20-98 years old.

DID YOU KNOW?

Unfortunately, McCullough found that women who gained weight after menopause did not experience the same degree of risk reduction when they exercised as women who maintained ideal body weight. It appears that weight gain, particularly after menopause, offsets the benefits provided by regular exercise.

What did the researchers discover about the benefits of exercise in this study?

Dr. Lauren McCullough, one of the investigators involved in the study, found that regular exercise reduced the risk for breast cancer in women of all ages and at all levels of physical activity. Her findings corroborated similar results reported in other peer-reviewed studies around the world.

What was the benefit of exercise in reducing the risk for breast cancer?

McCullough found that all levels and durations of exercise reduced the risk for breast cancer, with the greatest benefit (30% reduction in risk) seen in women who exercised 10-19 hours per week.

Did exercise reduce the risk for all types of breast cancer?

Yes, regular exercise reduced the risk for all types of breast cancer, especially estrogen-positive tumors which are the most common type of tumor in post-menopausal women in the United States.

Regular exercise has been proven to reduce the risk for breast cancer. The greatest risk reduction is seen in women who exercise moderately for 10-19 hours per week and who maintain ideal body weight throughout their lifetime. Even women as old as 98 can reduce their risk of breast cancer by including regular exercise, even modest exercise, into their daily routine.

Two B Vitamins Can Reduce the Risk for Breast Cancer in Women Who Drink Alcohol

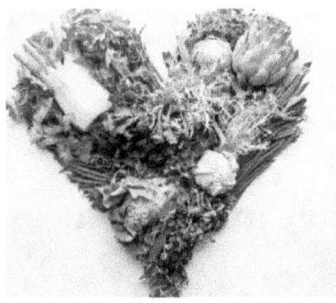

Drinking alcohol has been shown to increase the risk for breast cancer. Even half a glass of wine per day elevates the risk. But drinking red wine has been shown to help fight heart disease. So what's a woman to do? Scientists have discovered that increasing the quantity of two vitamins, folate and B6, can ameliorate the increased risk for breast cancer associated with alcohol consumption.

Folate

Folate is a form of folic acid, a substance found in leafy green vegetables and whole grains. It is one of the B vitamins and is considered necessary for a healthy diet.

Vitamin B6

Vitamin B6 is a water-soluble vitamin necessary for the normal function of many biochemical processes in the body. It is found in meats, whole grains, nuts, many vegetables and bananas.

DID YOU KNOW?

A Nurses Health Study looked at breast cancer risk among 712 women with breast cancer and 712 matched controls (similar women who did not have breast cancer.) Women with the highest folate levels had a 27% reduction in breast cancer risk compared to women with the lowest levels. Researchers then looked at only those women who drank one glass of wine or other alcoholic drink per day and found that high folate levels in these women reduced their risk of breast cancer by 89%. The researchers also found that women with the highest levels of vitamin B6 had a 30% lower risk for breast cancer. It seemed that folate and vitamin B6 had the greatest for reducing the risk for breast cancer in women who drank alcohol in moderation.

A glass of wine a day may be good for your heart but it will certainly increase your risk for breast cancer. To attenuate the risk make sure your diet is high in foods that contain folate and vitamin B6: leafy green vegetables, bananas, nuts, whole grains, and meat. Taking a daily multivitamin may also be a smart strategy to reduce the risk for breast cancer imparted by moderate alcohol consumption.

Breast Healthy Recipe: Broccoli with Anchovy and Garlic

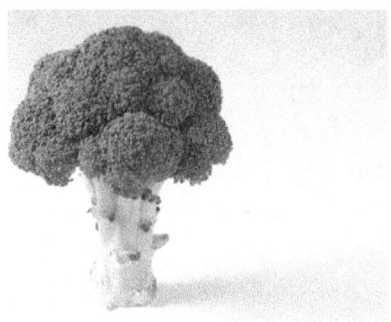

Cruciferous vegetables such as broccoli, cauliflower, brussels sprouts, and cabbage contain phytochemicals (e.g., isothiocyanates and indoles) that have been shown to protect against a variety of cancers. A recent study of 4800 breast cancer survivors diagnosed with Stage I-IV tumors between 2002 - 2006 found that women who ate cruciferous vegetables had a reduced risk for breast cancer recurrence and death. The observed benefit was dose-dependent; that is, women whose diets were highest in cruciferous vegetables derived the greatest protective benefit, achieving as much as a 62% reduction in breast cancer mortality during the first three years after diagnosis.

PREP TIME: 10 minutes

COOK TIME: 15 minutes

READY IN: 25 minutes

Ingredients

1 c - broccoli

1 - anchovy

1 tsp - garlic

1 tbsp - olive oil

Directions

Wash and trim the stems from the broccoli and separate florets into smaller pieces. Bring 2 quarts of water to a boil in a large pot and cook the broccoli for 5 minutes; then drain in a colander. Peel and finely chop the garlic. Heat the olive oil in a small saute pan over medium heat and add one anchovy fillet and the chopped garlic, mashing the anchovy together with the garlic and stirring for 2 minutes. Add the broccoli to the saute pan with the garlic and anchovy and toss and stir for another 2 minutes. Remove from heat and serve hot.

A diet high in cruciferous vegetables (broccoli, cauliflower, brussels sprouts, cabbage, and arugula) is associated with a reduced risk of breast cancer recurrence and death. Cruciferous vegetables contain phytochemicals such as isothiocyanates and indoles that appear to significantly improve outcomes in women diagnosed with Stage I-IV breast cancer, reducing the risk of death by as much as 62% in women whose diets are highest in these vegetables.

DID YOU KNOW?

Arugula is also a cruciferous vegetable, available in most markets year round, and can be added to salads to boost the dietary intake of phytochemicals.

The Best Foods to Eat During the Fall

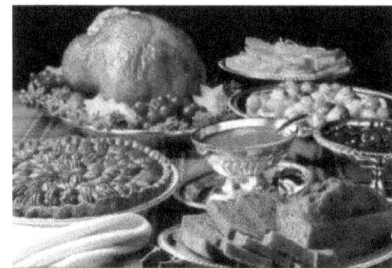

The fall season is going strong. We are moving closer and closer to Halloween and will be enjoying a delicious Thanksgiving dinner with our close friends and family in no time. Many families have gone on seasonal hayrides and apple picking adventures. Some have picked up pumpkins in their nearby orchards.

The autumn seems to have a multitude of delicious foods to pick from. However, it is important to pick the healthiest foods instead of solely fat- and sugar-filled meals. A healthy plant-based diet will help you stay trim and prevent a multitude of conditions including heart disease and breast cancer. As such, we will outline the type of produce and meals you would benefit from this autumn.

1. **Apples.** Make sure to spend some time apple picking this season! Apples are a great source of antioxidants and are full of fiber - they have four grams of dietary fiber per serving. Additionally, this fruit has flavonoids that keep your cardiovascular system functioning well. Whether you eat it raw or make applesauce, make sure to include this food in your diet over the next few months.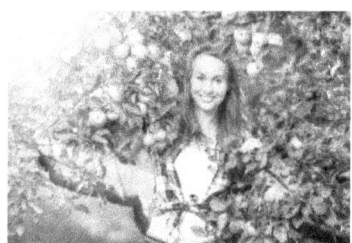

2. **Brussels sprouts.** If you're looking for a great addition to your dinner tonight, boil some Brussels sprouts and pan-fry them with some garlic - it'll taste delicious and pack a real vitamin K punch! The vegetable also has plenty of folate and iron.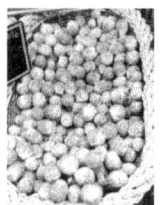

3. **Pears.** Along with apples, the fall brings us the harvest of pears. When cooking this fruit, try baking it or poaching it to really bring out the flavors. Pears are full of vitamin C, copper, and fiber.

4. **Butternut squash.** One of the most delicious foods you will find this season is the butternut squash. It is the perfect vegetable to make a sweet soup on those cooler, dreary days. Add some cinnamon and ginger when cooking squash to bring out some delicious flavors. Squash contains vitamin A and omega-3 fatty acids, which are known to prevent cancer.

5. **Pumpkin.** With Halloween right around the corner, the pumpkin is one type of produce that can be used for both decoration and your next meal! The pumpkin

has a sweet taste that makes it perfect for making pudding, pies, and cakes. Some of the basic health benefits of the pumpkin includes its rich source of potassium, fiber, and B vitamins.

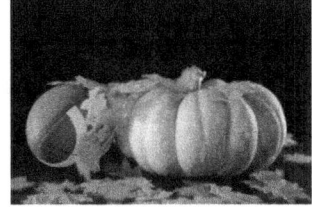

After you've gone to the market and stuffed your fridge with the above healthy foods, the next step to take is to find some great recipes and cook up a delicious meal. Looking to use those Brussels sprouts? Try this Roasted Brussels Sprouts With Crispy Capers and Carrots recipe.

After an afternoon of apple picking, are you looking for the best use for this fruit? Why not try this Rosemary-Apple Bread recipe? It's sure to blow the socks off your family! And how can you incorporate the rest of that butternut squash after you've already made your soup? Try your hand at this Ginger Butternut Squash and Tofu Curry dish!

For more tips on the best foods to incorporate in your diet, check out our articles below!

1. Breast Healthy Recipe: Chocolate Covered Brazil Nuts

2. Breast Healthy Recipe: Carrot Curry

3. Breast Healthy Recipe: Roasted Brussels Sprouts

4. Five Foods that Keep Your Breasts Healthy

Exercise and Lymphedema

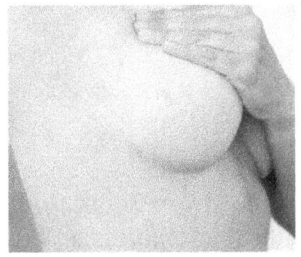

Breast cancer is terrifying. And, for the one in every eight women who will be diagnosed with it at some point in her life, anything that could prevent complications as a result of breast cancer is worth knowing about. Lymphedema, or obstruction of the lymph nodes resulting in swelling of the arms or legs, often comes about as the result of a mastectomy, adding insult to injury. The good news is that, if you do some special exercises, post-mastectomy lymphedema may be prevented entirely or, if it does occur, improved. Follow these simple tips.

Talk to a Specialist before Beginning

Anyone who has lymphedema or is at risk of lymphedema should talk to a specialized physician before beginning any exercise regimen as treatment. He or she will be able to tell you what will work best in your situation, and ensure that you know what you are doing before you begin.

Wear a Pressure Garment

If you have lymphedema and are doing exercises to help it, you should wear a pressure garment on the affected area. So, for those undertaking exercises after a mastectomy, a well-fitting compression bra and top may be a good choice. This ensures your safety and the maximum effectiveness of your exercises.

DID YOU KNOW?

Sometimes lymphedema that is the result of cancer treatment can show up years after the treatment has ended.

Begin with Light Weight Lifting

In women who have lymphedema as a result of a mastectomy, light upper-body exercises such as weight lifting can stop the progression of or even improve symptoms of lymphedema.

Work Your Way Up

When beginning your exercise regimen, begin with very light exercises. In time, you should gradually increase intensity, but keep in mind that if you stop exercising for a period of time of a week or longer, you should begin again at the lowest level. Do not overload your body.

If Symptoms Change, Consult Your Doctor

If you notice persistent changes that last a week or more, such as increased swelling of a limb or a sense of heaviness, you should talk to an expert in lymphedema exercises. He or she will be able to determine whether or not you should continue.

Consider Aerobic Activities

Aerobic activities such as jogging or swimming make your heart and lungs work harder, which in turn helps lymph nodes to push more lymph out of the affected area, creating less swelling. Be careful, however, and know your limits in this as in all other areas.

Don't Neglect Your Breathing

Though it may seem too simple, doing breathing exercises can also help expel lymph from your affected areas. Deep breathing and neck rolls are just a few simple exercises you can do to help in this area.

When you've already survived breast cancer, having to deal with yet another disease can be incredibly discouraging, if you let it be. Yet, with these simple lymphedema exercises, you can be master of your situation once again. Lymphedema can be treated, and its treatment is simple and effective. Just follow these tips, and you will find yourself well on the way to a more comfortable, and healthier, you.

Green Vegetables and Other Ways to Prevent Cancer

We are on our last days of October, a month dedicated to breast cancer awareness. The country seems to be awash in pink, but few are truly talking about the importance of breast cancer prevention. We need to spend more time focused on stopping this disease from affecting the women around us.

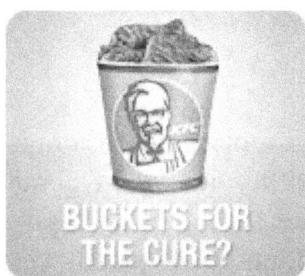

Ingrid Newkirk, founder of PETA, wrote for the Huffington Post that one of the best ways to prevent breast cancer is by following a healthy, plant-based diet. The Susan G. Komen Foundation, for instance, seems to bypass the importance of diet in cancer prevention, as the organization has previously partnered with Kentucky Fried Chicken through its "Buckets for the Cure" campaign. Red Baron Pizza has also apparently chosen a pink promotion to increase breast cancer ... I mean, breast cancer awareness. There are countless of studies that have found a high consumption of animal fat leads to a rise in breast cancer risk.

As such, it is ever so important to incorporate fruits, vegetables, and low-calorie produce in one's diet. Vegetarian diets have actually been associated with a low or reduced risk of cancer. In fact, Newkirk goes on to quote a study that says vegetarians are 40 percent less likely to be diagnosed with cancer as compared to those who eat meat. Another study found that, out of 35,000 women 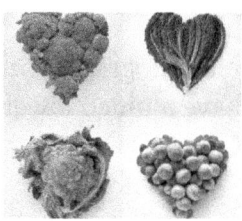 followed, the ones who had the highest consumption of meat also had the highest risk of breast cancer.

Plant foods have the highest amount of cancer-fighting antioxidants. For example, the antioxidant sulforaphane is found in broccoli, kale, cauliflower, and Brussels sprouts. Tomatoes have lycopene, which slows down cancer cell growth. Berries like blueberries have compounds that starve cancerous cells. Carrots and pumpkin as well as other colorful fruits are full of beta carotene, which also reduces breast cancer risk. Adding lentils, beans, whole grains, and walnuts in one's diet is also beneficial for overall health.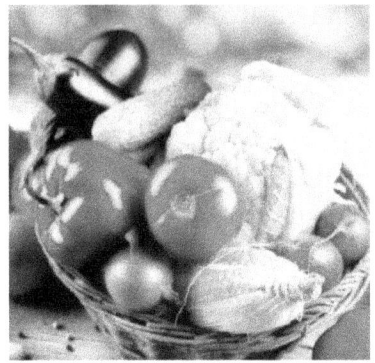

Prevention Magazine also emphasizes the importance of fitness when it comes to stopping breast cancer. Exercise helps one control weight, which is important in preventing obesity (a common risk factor for breast cancer). Physical activity has also shown to change estrogen metabolism. Women who go for a brisk walk for as little as two hours per week have an 18 percent lower risk of breast cancer when compared to women who are completely inactive, according to one study.

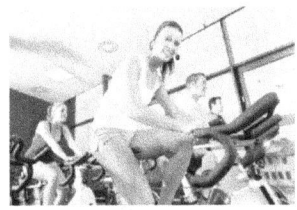

Other ways to prevent breast cancer is to avoid or stop hormone replacement therapy (HRT). These pills have been classified as carcinogenic. Talk with your doctor about other methods for solving any menopausal symptoms. If you are a mother and have recently given birth, consider breastfeeding your child. One study found that women who consistently breastfeed their child for the first six months after giving birth have a 10 percent lower risk of breast cancer mortality.

Also, if you are at high risk of breast cancer due to genetic mutations and/or family history, consider taking chemopreventive drugs like tamoxifen and increasing mammography screening to every six months. These solutions will lead any woman to have a much lower risk of breast cancer - something we should all focus on during Breast Cancer Awareness Month.

Surgical Options for Women with BRCA Mutations

Approximately 10% of breast cancer cases diagnosed in the United States are associated with a genetic, inherited predisposition to the disease. Of these patients, the majority carry a mutation in one of two genes, BRCA 1 and BRCA 2. These mutations are inherited from either parent and are passed to children in the same manner as, say, eye color. There are a variety of mutations that may occur on the BRCA genes, and all are associated with a range of increased risk for several cancers, including breast, ovarian, pancreatic, colon, and (in male carriers) prostate.

Women who carry a BRCA mutation are at an especially high lifetime risk for breast and ovarian cancer. Surgical removal of the breasts and ovaries reduces the risk and mortality associated with these tumors, but does not completely eradicate it because residual cells that harbor the BRCA mutation are invariable left behind and still retain the potential to produce tumors. Given below are current estimates of the value of surgical interventions aimed at reducing the risk for breast and ovarian cancer incidence and mortality in women who carry a BRCA mutation.

How significant is the risk of breast or ovarian cancer in women who carry a BRCA mutation?

Women who carry a BRCA mutation are at a 5-20 fold increased risk of developing breast or ovarian cancer. The risk for these tumors is somewhat broad because there is a variety of mutations that can occur, each with its own specific risk profile. In addition, other known risk factors for breast cancer, such as use of oral contraceptives, smoking, and alcohol ingestion, can interact with the BRCA mutation to increase the overall risk for malignancy.

What is the preventive benefit of prophylactic mastectomy in BRCA carriers?

On average, women who carry a BRCA mutation can expect to have a 90% reduction in their risk for breast cancer if they have their breasts removed. Risk reduction does not achieve 100% efficacy because even during the most thorough mastectomy, some BRCA mutated cells are invariably left behind such that a small, but significant, risk for breast cancer persists.

DID YOU KNOW?

Some women may elect an aggressive breast cancer screening program as an alternative to prophylactic mastectomy. An annual mammogram and an annual breast MRI, staggered so that one of each screening method is performed every six months, yields a survival benefit that approaches 95% of that achieved by prophylactic mastectomy. For this reason, many women choose prophylactic removal of the ovaries, which reduces the risk of breast cancer by 50%, and aggressive screening with mammogram and breast MRI rather than surgical removal of the breasts.

What is the preventive benefit of prophylactic ovary removal in BRCA carriers?

Prophylactic removal of the ovaries can reduce the risk of ovarian cancer in BRCA carriers by as much as 85% if it is performed before age 50. Because the risk of ovarian cancer in BRCA carriers increases every year as they get older, the greatest survival benefit is achieved if the ovaries are removed prior to menopause, preferably as soon as childbearing is complete.

Is there any other benefit of prophylactic removal of the ovaries in BRCA carriers?

Yes, removal of the ovaries by age 50 reduces the risk for breast cancer approximately 50%. The reason removing the ovaries lowers breast cancer risk is that breast cancer is, in large part, dependent on the presence of estrogen for growth and development. This is why removing the source of estrogen made by the ovaries serves to cut the risk for breast cancer in half.

What is the most successful surgical intervention to improve survival in BRCA carriers?

At this time, the most successful surgical intervention to improve survival in women who carry a BRCA mutation is a combined prophylactic mastectomy and removal of the ovaries. The best overall survival benefit is found in women who have a prophylactic mastectomy by age 25 and a prophylactic removal of the ovaries by age 40. BRCA carriers who chose this combined surgical prophylaxis can achieve an overall survival that approaches normal; that is, a survival that is similar to women who do not carry a BRCA mutation.

Women who inherit a mutation in BRCA genes are at an increased risk for breast, ovarian, pancreatic, and colon cancer. Surgical removal of the breasts can reduce the risk for breast cancer by as much as 90%. Surgical removal of the ovaries can reduce the risk for ovarian cancer by 85% and the risk of breast cancer by 50%. Because the risk for breast and ovarian cancer in BRCA carriers increases significantly every year of their life, it is generally recommended that prophylactic surgical procedures be offered to these women between the ages of 25-50 to maximize the preventive benefit of these risk reduction strategies.

Relief for the Pain of Breast Cancer

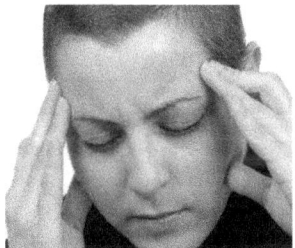

Dealing with painful breast cancer is something no one should have to do. However, if you find yourself in this position, it's important to realize that you do have options. As you fight your breast cancer, you can fight your pain, too. By looking into your options, and keeping in mind a few simple tips, you can relieve your discomfort. Dealing with breast cancer is difficult but you can certainly do something about the pain.

Talk to Your Doctor

Be sure to keep your doctor informed of any changes in your pain level. He or she will be able to provide you with expert advice and prescriptions as needed, and will know when your pain is a symptom that needs to be further explored.

Consider Over-the-Counter Options

Oftentimes, breast pain can be decreased dramatically by the use of over-the-counter painkillers such as acetaminophen (Tylenol) or aspirin. Be sure to consult your doctor before turning to these regularly, but keep in mind that over-the-counter drugs can provide a lot of relief without the side effects or the cost of a prescription painkiller.

EDITOR'S TIP:

Keep a journal of your pain level, so as to track how well your treatments are working and to provide your physician with information about your health.

Look into Home Remedies

Simple tricks like wearing a well-fitted bra, eating well, avoiding caffeine, and using cold and hot compresses can help alleviate breast pain. Remember that pain prevention doesn't have to be complicated, and that it can be cut down significantly by adjusting a few little things at home.

Consider Alternative Treatments

Many people find that holistic health treatments like massage, yoga, music, or acupuncture help their pain levels. Look around your neighborhood and see if these options exist near you, and spend some time focusing on making your whole body healthy and relaxed, in order to help cut down on your pain.

Don't Neglect Your Emotional Needs

The pain of breast cancer is never simply physical. Make sure you are taking care of your emotional self, as well. Find someone to talk to about it, and make sure you stay honest with yourself about how you are feeling and what you need.

Having painful breast cancer is difficult. However, for those in the know, it is possible to reduce the level of pain you are experiencing. Breast pain can be debilitating, or it can be manageable. Just a few tips can mean all the difference.

November 2014

Turkey, Stuffing, and Pumpkin Pie - Is it Possible to Stay Healthy during the Holidays?

We've moved forward into November and we all know that means Thanksgiving is right around the corner. Many families spend weeks preparing for this holiday. The cooks in each family buy turkeys ahead of time and begin prepping the food days before. Others are responsible for decorating the house and setting the table with centerpieces and tableware.

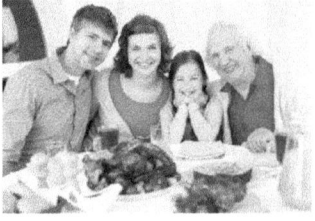

After playing a game of touch football, families throughout the United States often sit down to a large meal that may last hours. From turkey, stuffing, and mashed potatoes to yams, cranberry sauce, and pumpkin pie, Americans tend to overeat on this holiday and may have difficulty sticking to a healthy diet.

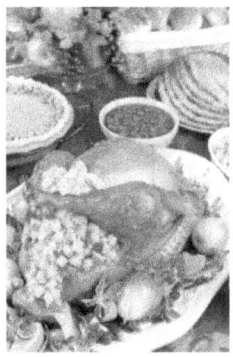

So if you are dedicated to remaining healthy regardless of the time of year, how do you stay healthy during the holidays? According to Reader's Digest, it is helpful to focus on other parts of the holiday instead of the food. Spend time talking with your family, laughing and telling jokes. Going for a walk or throwing around a football is also encouraged.

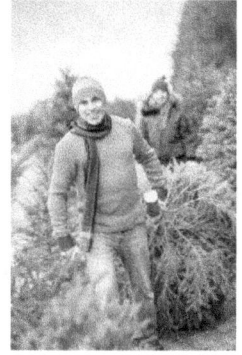

One way to avoid overeating during the large Thanksgiving meal is to not skip breakfast. Have some cereal, whole-grain toast, and fruit. Another way to burn some extra calories is to cut down your own Christmas tree soon after Thanksgiving. Walking around a tree farm will give you great memories with your family and allow you to burn off that turkey stuffing or extra bread roll.

When you sit down to eat dinner on Thanksgiving day, have some salad to start. That will fill you up partially, so that you won't overeat on the unhealthier items. Be sure to stick to only your absolute favorite foods and avoid the extra - that will also keep the calories down.

If you love turkey, gravy and cranberry sauce, stick to these foods and don't put a mound of mashed potatoes on that plate. When pouring sauces or gravy over your food, stick to a small amount. Additionally, stick to only one or two glasses of wine on Thanksgiving. There is no need to indulge in alcohol on a joyous family occasion.

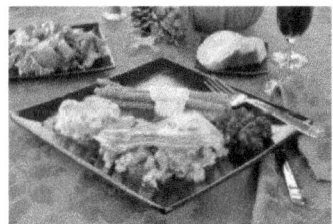

Be sure to keep healthy meals in your freezer throughout December, so that you won't be stuck going out to a fast food joint for your dinners. Be sure to incorporate fruits and vegetables in your diet. If you are bringing a dish to Thanksgiving or cooking the meal yourself, try to follow healthy recipes that are lower in fat.

Staying physically active throughout the holidays is also extremely important, as it will keep you from gaining unwanted weight. One blog post encourages you to set an exercise schedule. Try to go on 15-minute walks twice a day. By following these tips, you'll be able to stay healthy on Thanksgiving day and the coming holidays.

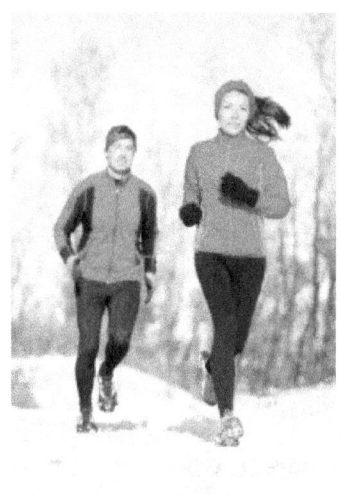

Much Ado about Radiation Therapy

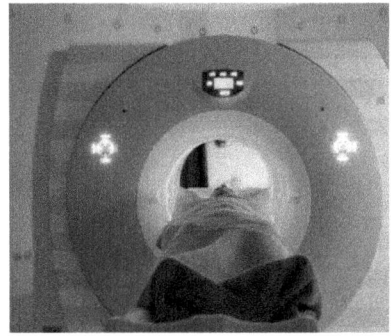

Nothing is perfect. Certainly, breast cancer treatment is no exception. We are saving lives and saving breasts, more than ever before. But saving breasts requires adjuvant radiation therapy; and though it is essential, it's far from perfect.

Why is radiation therapy required for breast-conservation?

Women who have lumpectomy (i.e., breast-conserving surgery) for early-stage breast cancers have an unacceptably high local recurrence rate if radiation therapy is not included as part of the treatment plan. The addition of radiation therapy reduces the risk of local recurrence to less than 1% per year, a very acceptable rate. Which is to say, about one woman in a hundred per year who undergoes lumpectomy followed by radiation therapy will have a local recurrence of breast cancer.

A study about the long-terms effects of radiation therapy in women with breast cancer was published in the New England Journal of Medicine on March 14, 2013. What did it show?

Researchers were concerned that breast cancer patients treated with lumpectomy followed by radiation therapy would have an increased risk for heart disease due to exposure of the heart muscle to extraneous radiation during therapy. They studied a population of women treated with radiation therapy for breast cancer between 1958 and 2001 in Sweden and Denmark, and recorded the incidence of heart attacks in these patients.

They compared the risk of heart attack to the amount of radiation each woman received as part of her treatment. They found what others had found previously: an increased incidence of heart attack associated with radiation therapy, proportional to the amount of radiation received.

The researchers also noted that the risk for heart attack increased rather quickly, within two years of treatment, and continued for at least 20 years thereafter. Not surprisingly, they also found that women with the highest pre-treatment risk factors for heart disease had the greatest risk of heart attack following radiation therapy for breast cancer.

Is there anything about this study that needs to be understood or explained other than the data presented in the paper?

Yes. It's important to appreciate the the manner in which radiation therapy was delivered forty years ago was much cruder and exposed the heart to far more radiation than is delivered today.

Are there any other benefits to radiation therapy besides reducing the risk of local recurrence of breast cancer?

Yes. A meta-analysis of 17 randomized trials comprising approximately 11,000 women showed that radiation therapy reduced the risk of death from breast cancer, even 15 years after treatment. Therefore, radiation therapy provides a survival benefit in addition to local control of disease.

There are approximately three million women breast cancer survivors living in the United States at this time. The majority have had radiation therapy as part of their treatment, and the majority have been able to keep their breasts and their lives free of additional recurrent disease. Radiation therapy has its risks, no doubt, but with modern modalities the risk of cardiac disease in women whose baseline risk is low remains low after treatment with breast-conservation and state of the art radiation therapy.

DID YOU KNOW?

State of the art radiation therapy using a linear accelerator, instead of the archaic cobalt 60 treatments used in the 1950's and 1960's, with attention to protection of the heart and lungs, today provides minimal exposure of the heart muscle to scatter radiation during breast cancer treatment.

Acupuncture and Exercise Relieves Symptoms in Breast Cancer Patients

Breast cancer treatment is never a pleasant experience. Radiation, surgery, or chemotherapy can all lead to significant pain and various other side effects. A new study, however, may have found a way to alleviate the pain and swelling associated with breast cancer treatments.

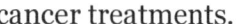

HealthDay News reported that acupuncture and exercise may bring relief to cancer patients who are experiencing pain. The results show that acupuncture relieved joint pain by as much as 40 percent. A placebo affect should not have occurred, as people's opinions on whether it would work or not did not seem to affect the outcome.

Previous research also shows how acupuncture can relieve fatigue, joint pain, and sleeping issues. Study author Dr. Jun Mao, director of the integrative oncology program at the Abramson Cancer Center at the University of Pennsylvania, followed 41 breast cancer patients and assigned them to three groups. The first two groups were a sham type of acupuncture and electroacupuncture while the third group received neither treatment and was considered a control group.

The women in the three groups had stiffness and joint pain, which are typical side effects from the hormonal therapy drugs aromatase inhibitors. The women in the electroacupuncture group had a persistent amount of pain reduction while no changes were reported in the sham group.

"The real acupuncture group, regardless of expectation, everyone had about a 40 percent reduction in pain," Mao told the news source. "Real acupuncture will work for anyone, whether you believe it or not."

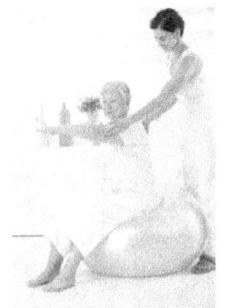

University of Pennsylvania researchers also took a look at how an exercise program can relieve lymphedema (a type of swelling) and muscle problems. The program was offered by physical therapists and patients were taught exercises to perform at home or at the gym. After one year, the patients had improved symptoms and stronger muscles.

Both physical fitness and acupuncture could benefit breast cancer patients and survivors that are suffering from side effects of treatment. If you are in pain, ask your doctor about an exercise program or an acupuncturist. It may help you get back to your old self!

The Role of Estrogen in Breast Tissue

Estrogen is a female sex hormone made by the ovaries and released into the bloodstream where it circulates throughout the body. It enters specific cells in the body that carry estrogen receptors, proteins that allow estrogen to enter the cell. The primary target for estrogen is the cells of the breast and cells that line the uterus, vagina, and cervix.

What role does estrogen play in the breast?

Estrogen is responsible for initial growth of the breast during puberty. It also maintains the normal function of the breast during the reproductive years, particularly cells that line the ducts of the breast.

What causes the ovaries to release estrogen?

The pituitary gland located in the center of the brain releases a hormone that causes the ovaries to manufacture and release estrogen into the bloodstream.

DID YOU KNOW?

The majority of breast cancers contain estrogen receptors. Just as estrogen causes normal breast cells to grow, breast cancer cells that carry estrogen receptors will also grow in the presence of estrogen. For this reason, women who have been diagnosed with breast cancer should not take drugs that contain estrogen such as hormone replacement therapy.

Why do estrogen levels fall after menopause?

After menopause, the ovaries can no longer make estrogen.

Estrogen is a hormone made by the ovaries in response to stimulation by the pituitary gland. Estrogen causes the breasts to grow during puberty and helps to maintain normal breast function during the reproductive years. After menopause the ovaries can no longer make estrogen and as a result estrogen levels fall significantly. The majority of breast cancers grow in the presence of estrogen; thus, women diagnosed with breast cancer should not take drugs that contain estrogen such as hormone replacement therapy.

Phase I Clinical Trial for Preventive Breast Cancer Vaccine Expected to Start in 2015!

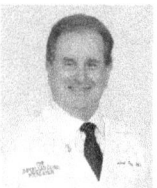

Major changes are occurring for the one and only preventive breast cancer vaccine of the Cleveland Clinic. This vaccine was found to prevent breast cancer on 100 percent of animal models studied and the research was published in the May 2010 issue of *Nature Medicine*. Ever since, study author Dr. Vincent Tuohy and his team have worked on gathering the funds necessary to begin Phase I clinical trials to see if the vaccine is as safe and effective in women as in mice.

After years of effort, finally the funding came through in September 2013 when anonymous private investors provided the money needed to start the next step of research. A spin-off company called Shield Biotech has been working ever since on gaining FDA approval to start trials, recruit subjects, and gather the resources necessary to get the research off the ground.

The Pink Paper explains that clinical trials for the preventive breast cancer vaccine are expected to start in 2015. These initial trials will work on determining the right dosage and determine the safety of the vaccine. It is predicted that this therapy can prevent the most lethal form of breast cancer called triple negative breast cancer. Initially, the women who will be subjects in the study will have already had triple negative breast cancer and the therapy will be used to prevent recurrence. A second phase of the trial will include women who have a high genetic risk of developing breast cancer. These will be women who also wish to undergo a mastectomy to prevent cancer. After the mastectomy, the tissues will be studied to see if the vaccine caused any inflammation or tissue damage. This part of the study will help analyze the safety of the vaccine.

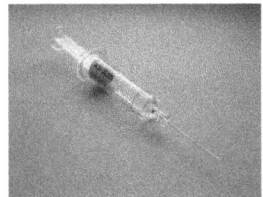

Phase I will take several years to complete. If all goes well, further studies will determine the overall efficacy of the vaccine. It may be ten or more years until we see whether this vaccine can go from bench to bedside. Nonetheless, this is very exciting news. We may see the results of a Phase I study in only a few years!

www.ingramcontent.com/pod-product-compliance
Lightning Source LLC
Chambersburg PA
CBHW081835170526
45167CB00007B/2814